T0321073

Nursing Leadership in Long-Term Care

Editors

MELODEE HARRIS
ANN KOLANOWSKI
SHERRY GREENBERG

NURSING CLINICS
OF NORTH AMERICA

www.nursing.theclinics.com

Consulting Editor
BENJAMIN SMALLHEER

June 2022 • Volume 57 • Number 2

ELSEVIER

1600 John F. Kennedy Boulevard • Suite 1800 • Philadelphia, Pennsylvania, 19103-2899

http://www.theclinics.com

NURSING CLINICS OF NORTH AMERICA Volume 57, Number 2
June 2022 ISSN 0029-6465, ISBN-13: 978-0-323-91996-8

Editor: Kerry Holland
Developmental Editor: Axell Ivan Jade M. Purificacion

Nursing Clinics of North America (ISSN 0029-6465) is published quarterly by Elsevier Inc., 360 Park Avenue South, New York, NY 10010-1710. Months of issue are March, June, September, and December. Periodicals postage paid at New York, NY and additional mailing offices. Subscription price per year is, $163.00 (US individuals), $689.00 (US institutions), $275.00 (international individuals), $710.00 (international institutions), $231.00 (Canadian individuals), $710.00 (Canadian institutions), $100.00 (US and Canadian students), and $135.00 (international students). To receive student/resident rate, orders must be accompanied by name of affiliated institution, date of term, and the signature of program/residency coordinator on institution letterhead. Orders will be billed at individual rate until proof of status is received. Foreign air speed delivery is included in all *Clinics* subscription prices. All prices are subject to change without notice. **POSTMASTER:** Send address changes to *Nursing Clinics*, Elsevier Health Sciences Division, Subscription Customer Service, 3251 Riverport Lane, Maryland Heights, MO 63043. **Customer Service: Telephone: 1-800-654-2452** (U.S. and Canada); **1-314-447-8871 (outside U.S. and Canada). Fax: 1-314-447-8029. E-mail: journalscustomerservice-usa@ elsevier.com** (for print support) and **journalsonlinesupport-usa@elsevier.com** (for online support).

Nursing Clinics of North America is covered in *EMBASE/Excerpta Medica, MEDLINE/PubMed (Index Medicus), Social Sciences Citation Index, Current Contents, ASCA, Cumulative Index to Nursing, RNdex Top 100,* and Allied Health Literature and International Nursing Index (INI).

Contributors

CONSULTING EDITOR

BENJAMIN SMALLHEER, PhD, RN, ACNP-BC, FNP-BC, CCRN, CNE
Associate Clinical Professor, School of Nursing, Duke University, Durham, North Carolina, USA

EDITORS

MELODEE HARRIS, PhD, RN, FAAN
Associate Professor, College of Nursing, University of Arkansas for Medical Sciences, Little Rock, Arkansas, USA

ANN KOLANOWSKI, PhD, RN, FAAN
Professor Emerita, Ross and Carol Nese College of Nursing, Penn State University, University Park, Pennsylvania, USA

SHERRY GREENBERG, PhD, RN, FAAN
Associate Professor, Seton Hall University, Nutley, New Jersey, USA

AUTHORS

DEB BAKERJIAN, PhD, APRN, FAAN, FAANP, FGSA
Clinical Professor, Betty Irene Moore School of Nursing, UC Davis, Sacramento, California, USA

ALICE BONNER, PhD, RN
Institute for Healthcare Improvement, Boston, Massachusetts, USA

PAMELA Z. CACCHIONE, PhD, CRNP, BC, FGSA, FAAN
Ralston House Term Chair in Gerontological Nursing, Professor of Geropsychiatric Nursing, Nurse Scientist at Penn Presbyterian Medical Center, University of Pennsylvania School of Nursing, Philadelphia, Pennsylvania, USA

TARA A. CORTES, PhD, RN, FAAN, FGSA
Executive Director and Clinical Professor, Hartford Institute for Geriatric Nursing at NYU Rory Meyers College of Nursing, New York, New York, USA

MARGARET DAWSON, LCSW
Silverado Senior Living, Los Angeles, California, USA

PAMELA B. DE CORDOVA, PhD, RN-BC
Associate Professor, Rutgers, The State University of New Jersey, School of Nursing, Newark, New Jersey, USA

MARY ELLEN DELLEFIELD, PhD, RN, FAAN
Adjunct Professor, Department of Community Health Systems, School of Nursing, University of California, San Francisco, San Francisco, California, USA

TERRY FULMER, PhD, RN
John A. Hartford Foundation, New York, New York, USA

DEANNA GRAY-MICELI, PhD, GNP-BC, FGSA, FAAN
Professor, Thomas Jefferson University, Jefferson College of Nursing, Philadelphia, Pennsylvania, USA

LAURIE GREALISH, RN, PhD, FACN
Associate Professor, Subacute and Aged Nursing, Deputy Higher Degrees Convener, Nursing and Midwifery, Menzies Health Institute Queensland, Griffith University and Nursing and Midwifery Education and Research Unit, Gold Coast Hospital and Health Services, Griffith University, Southport, Queensland, Australia

SHERRY GREENBERG, PhD, RN, FAAN
Associate Professor, Seton Hall University, Nutley, New Jersey, USA

MELODEE HARRIS, PhD, RN, APRN, FAAN
Associate Professor, College of Nursing, University of Arkansas for Medical Sciences, Little Rock, Arkansas, USA

ANN KOLANOWSKI, PhD, RN, FAAN
Professor Emerita, Ross and Carol Nese College of Nursing, Penn State University, University Park, Pennsylvania, USA

ALISON E. KRIS, PhD, RN, FGSA
Professor, Marion Peckham Egan School of Nursing, Fairfield University, Fairfield, Connecticut, USA

PAMELA LABORDE, DNP, APRN, CCNS
Clinical Assistant Professor, University of Arkansas for Medical Sciences, College of Nursing, Arkansas, Little Rock, Arkansas, USA

RUTH PALAN LOPEZ, PhD, GNP-BC, FGSA, FAAN
Associate Dean for Research School of Nursing, Jacques Mohr Endowed Professor, Gerontological Nursing, MGH Institute of Health Professions, MGH Institute of Health Professions School of Nursing, Boston, Massachusetts, USA

CAROLINE MADRIGAL, PhD, RN
Center of Innovation in Long-term Services and Supports, Providence VA Medical Center, Providence, Rhode Island, USA

ANN M. MAYO, RN, DNSc, FAAN
Hahn School of Nursing and Health Science, Beyster Institute of Nursing Research, University of San Diego, San Diego, California, USA

CHRISTINE MUELLER, PhD, RN, FGSA, FAAN
Long-term Care Professorship in Nursing, University of Minnesota, School of Nursing, Minneapolis, Minnesota, USA

ADRIA E. NAVARRO, PhD, LCSW
Associate Professor, Department of Social Work, Azusa Pacific University, Azusa, California, USA

LESLIE PELTON, MPA
Institute for Healthcare Improvement, Boston, Massachusetts, USA

MARINA RENTON, MPhil
Institute for Healthcare Improvement, Boston, Massachusetts, USA

KATHY RICHARDS, PhD, RN, FAAN, FAASM
Research Professor and Senior Scientist, School of Nursing, University of Texas at Austin, Austin, Texas, USA

JEANNETTE A. ROGOWSKI, PhD
Professor of Health Policy and Administration, The Pennsylvania State University, University Park, Pennsylvania, USA

SARAH C. ROSSMASSLER, DNP, AGPCNP-BC, ANP-BC, ACHPN
Assistant Professor, MGH Institute of Health Professions School of Nursing, Boston, Massachusetts, USA

STACY SHIPWAY, MSN, PHN, DNP(c)
Doctoral Student, Azusa Pacific University, School of Nursing, Azusa, California, USA

WANDA SPURLOCK, DNS, RN, GERO-BC, PMH-BC, CNE, FNGNA, ANEF, FAAN
Professor, College of Nursing and Allied Health, Southern University and A&M College, Baton Rouge, Louisiana, USA

DIANA LYNN WOODS, PhD, RN, APRN-BC, FGSA, FAAN
Professor, Department of Doctoral Programs, School of Nursing, Azusa Pacific University, Azusa, California, USA

Contents

Nurse leaders are first and foremost, registered nurses. Nursing leadership is critical for improving the care and quality of life for older adults. Visionary nurse leaders collaborate, motivate, influence, and inspire the achievement of values and goals to improve the quality of life for older adults in long-term care. Professional registered nurses are transformational servant nurse leaders who hold the key to nursing home reform.

Nurse staffing involves determining, allocating, and delivering nursing resources and care to residents in order to achieve the desired and required quality of care and life for residents. A comprehensive evidence-based framework for nurse staffing in nursing homes is presented to be considered beyond the number of nurse staff and consequently the nurse staffing strategies needed to address care quality in nursing homes.

Age-Friendly Health Systems Is a movement to ensure that all care and support for and with older adults across all settings is age-friendly care. Age-Friendly Health Systems provide staff, leadership, and care partner education based on the 4M Framework (What Matters, Medications, Mentation, Mobility). Nursing homes and other settings are often left out of local, state, or federal strategic plans on aging. In addition, limited quality and quantity of nursing home staff impact new program implementation. We consider how programs and services to support older adults can create and sustain an Age-Friendly Ecosystem, including a meaningful role for nursing homes.

This article focuses on factors contributing to the state of long-term care in this country. It highlights federal legislation which delegated much oversight to the states resulting in the lack of uniform standards for leadership qualifications, staffing levels, and payment. It describes how existing payment models and hierarchical leadership styles contribute to the system's inability to recruit and retain qualified staff and the need for education to prepare nurses and direct caregivers to work with the complex population in today's nursing homes.

Enhanced dementia-specific nursing care is needed to incorporate the rapid changes in dementia science for an expanding population of persons living with dementia (PLWD) in long-term care. Dementia-specific nursing care competencies should be incorporated into current curricula for undergraduate and graduate nursing programs as well as nurse professional practice. This article proposes a set of dementia nursing care competencies that reflect current scientific findings on neurodegenerative dementia diseases, communication and shared decision-making, supportive care management for symptoms of distress and deficits in activities of daily living, risk assessments for adverse outcomes, palliative care and advance directives, and caregiver issues.

Geropsychiatric nursing (GPN) leaders in long-term care settings have a 25-year tradition of innovation that has strikingly improved mental health and quality of life for older adult residents. The impact of the Coronavirus disease of 2019 (COVID-19) on the mental health of older adult residents and today's evolving health care systems requires additional GPN leaders well-prepared to advocate, plan, and deliver care for this vulnerable population. In this article, the authors discuss GPN leadership in the context of its history, the role of professional organizations, and educational competencies. A leadership exemplar is provided as well as recommendations for clinical practice and research.

This article highlights the critical role of advanced practice registered nurses in the care of older adults living in nursing homes. This population is one of the frailest, marginalized, and often neglected in the United States. The COVID-19 pandemic impact on nursing homes resulted in a stunning number of infections and subsequent resident deaths. This is a shameful reminder of the many challenges and gaps in the nursing home industry including inadequate staffing, high staff turnover, improper isolation technique, and lack of fundamental knowledge of how to adequately implement infection prevention and control processes. Strong advanced practice registered nurse leadership may have mitigated some of these factors.

Alzheimer disease and related dementias (ADRD) are irreversible, progressive brain disorders. Many people with ADRD experience the final stage of the disease, advanced dementia, in nursing homes (NHs). Although palliative care, including symptom management and emotional support for caregivers, is advocated for those with advanced dementia, many NH residents experience potentially burdensome interventions, such as feeding tubes, hospital transfers, and intensive rehabilitation. Nurses play a critical role in ensuring high-quality palliative care to residents with advanced dementia. The aim of this article is to raise awareness of the palliative care needs of NH residents with advanced dementia.

Nursing leaders have a responsibility to promote and facilitate social engagement and connectedness to mitigate social isolation in long-term care (LTC). The COVID-19 pandemic has emphasized longstanding problems in LTC facilities, such as staff mix, workload, and support. The pandemic has shed light on the severe deleterious effect of social isolation and the critical importance of maintaining social engagement and connectedness, especially in times of crisis or major change. Staff education and ongoing support cannot be overemphasized. Critical nursing leadership and interdisciplinary collaboration engaging all team members are essential in operationalizing nonpharmacological approaches that foster the well-being of residents with dementia.

Protecting frail older residents from adverse health outcomes associated with preventable illnesses and conditions, such as geriatric syndromes within the long-term care (LTC) health system requires attention by the health care team, led by professional nurse leaders, to all of the operant contextual factors influencing health outcomes. Mitchell's Health Outcomes Model helps to frame these operant contextual factors to help understand how the person and the situation are viewed, which then directs professional nurse leaders' interventions. Utilization of the LTC facilities Quality Metrics data can shape and inform nurses leaders as to the gaps which can be filled to meet resident care needs operant among these modifiable contextual factors.

The work environment is a modifiable construct associated with the quality of nursing home care. This article describes and explains variables known to be associated with the work environment of nurses in nursing homes, including the history and characteristics of nursing homes; the nature of nursing work; the nursing skill mix, and care delivery. Nursing leadership has the potential to transform the nursing home work environment and improve quality of care through education, research, advocacy, and implementation of evidence-based practices.

NURSING CLINICS

SERIES OF RELATED INTEREST

Critical Care Nursing Clinics of North America
https://www.ccnursing.theclinics.com/
Advances in Family Practice Nursing
www.advancesinfamilypracticenursing.com

THE CLINICS ARE AVAILABLE ONLINE!
Access your subscription at:
www.theclinics.com

Foreword

The Art of Nursing Leadership in a Challenging Patient Care Environment

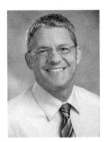

Benjamin Smallheer, PhD, RN, ACNP-BC, FNP-BC, CCRN, CNE
Consulting Editor

Long-term care is often thought to encompass the final stages of life for our aging and older adult population. The National Institute on Aging (2017)[1] describes the intent of long-term care as meeting a person's health and personal care needs through a variety of services. The goal of this specialized patient care is to help individuals live as independently and safely as possible when day-to-day activities have become challenging.

The phrase "long-term care" may bring the mental visualization of a nursing home or assisted living facility. Once in the facility, the person may receive assistance with toileting, bathing, dressing, grooming, and eating. All of these constitute "activities of daily living." Long-term care also extends to adult daycare centers, community centers, transportation services, and meal preparation and delivery with a significant quantity of care often provided by unlicensed health care providers: the individual's family members and loved ones.

The focus of attention is on the patient and their lived experience. However, there is an alternative side to the long-term care environment...the nursing side. The specialized care given to the older adult patient may be directed and/or provided by a certified nursing assistant, a licensed practical nurse, a registered nurse, or an advanced practice registered nurse. These nurses must deliver high-quality care to a patient population needing support for conditions such as dementia, debilitation, frailty, and palliative care. Serving as a nursing leader in such an environment requires an art not taught in the academic setting.

Nursing leadership in long-term care spans significant breadth, diversity, and environments outside of what is often considered nursing. It extends into the patient's homes, among their family, and into the community. The challenges encountered by nurse leaders in the long-term care environment are unique and include leadership

https://doi.org/10.1016/j.cnur.2022.03.002
0029-6465/22/© 2022 Published by Elsevier Inc.
nursing.theclinics.com

development and sustainability, health care reform and reimbursement, geropsychiatric complexities, social isolation, and societal expectations of health outcomes. All of these must be continually appraised and readdressed in ways that are specific to the long-term care environment.

This issue, dedicated to the tireless efforts of the nursing leadership in long-term care, provides a unique perspective on not just the challenges facing nursing leadership in long-term care but also success strategies that can get nurse leaders to the next level.

Benjamin Smallheer, PhD, RN, ACNP-BC, FNP-BC, CCRN, CNE
Duke University School of Nursing
307 Trent Drive
Box 3322, Office 3117
Durham, NC 27710, USA

E-mail address:
benjamin.smallheer@duke.edu

REFERENCE

1. National Institute on Aging. What is long-term care?. 2017. Available at: https://www.nia.nih.gov/health/what-long-term-care.

Preface

Overview of Nurse Leadership

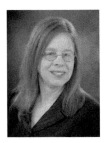 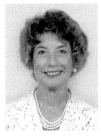 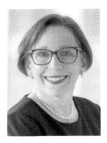

Melodee Harris,
PhD, RN, FAAN

Ann Kolanowski,
PhD, RN, FAAN
Editors

Sherry Greenberg,
PhD, RN, FAAN

As the largest and most trusted health care discipline, nurses are uniquely positioned to provide leadership in the delivery of quality care. Nowhere is this more obvious than in long-term care settings that service the growing population of older adults. Long-term care settings are places where nursing skills and interests are particularly well matched with residents' needs.[1] They are also settings where there is enormous potential for nurses to innovate and implement models of professional practice that successfully integrate these settings into the mainstream of health care.[2] Until recently, however, the relevance of strong nursing leadership to quality long-term care had too often been an unrecognized, unappreciated, and untapped resource in the industry. There is ample evidence that investment in professional nursing leadership is essential to the health and well-being of our nation's most vulnerable older adults.[3]

Over a decade ago, *Nursing Clinics of North America*[4] published an issue that focused exclusively on long-term care. In that series of articles, long-standing challenges to the delivery of quality care were discussed, and potential solutions were proposed. What is most striking is that many of these same challenges persist today: inadequate staffing levels, lack of clinical leadership, and health care disparities. What is changing is the overwhelming public endorsement for greater governmental funding and resources for long-term care similar to those in the acute care sector.[5] Most instrumental in the growing momentum for change has been the devasting effects of a pandemic, which were exacerbated in facilities that lacked a strong presence of professional nurse leadership.[6] These heart-wrenching stories, indeed much of what we read in the media, portray long-term care settings as places of last resort, avoided at all costs not only by older adults but also by the very people who could make a difference, professional nurse leaders.

This issue of *Nursing Clinics of North America* brings together articles authored by leading gerontological nursing scholars who, together, provide a vision of what high-quality long-term care is and the policy changes necessary to make it a reality.

Nurs Clin N Am 57 (2022) xv–xvii
https://doi.org/10.1016/j.cnur.2022.03.001
0029-6465/22/© 2022 Published by Elsevier Inc.

nursing.theclinics.com

These gerontological nurse leaders tell us that long-term care settings have much to offer older adults and are exciting places to work when nurses have the autonomy to exercise professional leadership. Several articles focus on the knowledge and competencies needed to care for residents who have complex health issues: those who are frail, mentally ill, socially isolated, at risk for/experiencing infection, or at end-of-life. Three articles describe transformative models of care that rely on and promote strong nursing leadership: The Advanced Practice Registered Nurse, Intraprofessional Practice, and Age-Friendly Care Models. There is also an article on the staffing levels required and retention efforts needed to help ensure the delivery of high-quality care.

A common underlying theme across the articles in this issue is that they all address, in one manner or another, how quality care can be achieved in nursing homes through *Transformational Leadership*.[7,8] One definition of nurse leadership is *inspiring and catalyzing others to achieve shared goals and institutional mission in an environment where the context and meanings are evolving, thus the constant need to design new ways of achieving long-held values.*[7] Transformational leaders use knowledge and skills to inspire, influence, and motivate staff to provide high-quality care.[8] Transformational leaders not only identify areas for improvement but also act upon and support team members toward common goals. Transformational leaders are proactive; they serve as a catalyst for innovation, and they create a learning environment so organizational realities are changed for the better. The articles in this issue support the development of transformative leaders.

Since 2020, there have been several commissions/panels that have been charged with improving and safeguarding the health and quality of life of residents who live in long-term care settings.[9] These efforts are laudable. For years gerontological nurse leaders have provided compelling evidence that supports the need for strong professional nurse presence in nursing homes.[10] Unfortunately, nursing leadership is most noticeable in its absence as we have seen over the past 2 years. As guest editors of this important issue, we feel the events occurring across the globe present an unprecedented opportunity to add the strong voice of expert nurse scientists, educators, and practitioners who, better than any discipline, understand how nursing leadership can transform long-term care.

Melodee Harris, PhD, RN, FAAN
University of Arkansas for Medical Sciences
4301 West Markham Street
Slot #529
Little Rock, AR 72205, USA

Ann Kolanowski, PhD, RN, FAAN
Ross and Carol Nese College of Nursing
Penn State University
University Park, PA 16802, USA

Sherry Greenberg, PhD, RN, FAAN
Seton Hall University
Nutley, NJ 07110, USA

E-mail addresses:
harrismelodee@uams.edu (M. Harris)
amk20@psu.edu (A. Kolanowski)
sherry.greenberg@shu.edu (S. Greenberg)

REFERENCES

1. Mezey MD, Mitty EL, Burger SG. Rethinking teaching nursing homes: potential for improving long-term care. Gerontologist 2008;48:8–15.
2. Siegel EO, Young HM. Assuring quality in nursing homes: the black box of administrative and clinical leadership—a scoping review. Gerontologist 2021;61: e147–62.
3. Bakerjian D, Boltz M, Bowers B, et al. Expert nurse response to workforce recommendations made by the coronavirus commission for safety and quality in nursing homes. Nurs Outlook 2021. https://doi.org/10.1016/j.outlook.2021.03.017. S0029-6554(21)00091-00099.
4. Dumas LG. Long-term care. Nurs Clin North Am 2009;44:161–270.
5. Brown D. Lawmakers want nursing home commission to include ombudsmen; study reveals public support for nursing homes. McKnight's Long-Term Care News; 2020. Available at: https://www.mcknights.com/news/lawmakers-want-nursinghome-commission-to-include-ombudsmen-study-revealspublic-support-for-nursing-homes.
6. Harrington C, Ross L, Chapman S, et al. Nurse staffing and coronavirus infections in California nursing homes. Policy Polit Nurs Pract 2020;21(3):174–86.
7. McBride A. The growth and development of nurse leaders. 2nd edition. Springer Publishing Co, LLC; 2020.
8. Broome ME, Marshall ES. Transformational leadership in nursing. 3rd edition. Springer Publishing Co; 2021.
9. National Academies of Sciences. Engineering and Medicine. Improving the quality of care in nursing homes. Washington, DC: The National Academies Press; 2021.
10. Kolanowski A, Horgas A, Wallhagen M, et al. A call to the CMS: mandate adequate professional nurse staffing in nursing homes. Am J Nurs 2020;121(3): 24–7.

The Making of Nurse Leaders in the Nursing Home

Melodee Harris, PhD, RN, FAAN[a],*, Ann Kolanowski, PhD, RN, FAAN[b],
Sherry Greenberg, PhD, RN, FAAN[c]

KEYWORDS

- Long-term care • Leadership • Transformational leadership • Servant leadership

KEY POINTS

- Nurse leaders are first and foremost, registered nurses.
- Nurse leaders in long-term care are change agents who anticipate continuously evolving policies, regulations, and priorities.
- The Future of Nursing Report supports that reforming health care for older adults is possible when regulation is placed into the hands of strong nursing leadership.

INTRODUCTION

Nurse leaders are made not born. One setting that cries out for nurse leaders is long-term care, a setting that has been in short supply of leadership for decades. This article reflects on what nursing leadership is, the educational and experiential paths that prepare nurse leaders, the characteristics and role of nurse leaders in long-term care, and recommendations for improving nursing leadership in long-term care settings. This overview is a background for the other articles in this special issue, all of which ultimately aim to improve the care of older adults who reside in long-term care settings.

There are several definitions of nurse leadership that apply to the professional nurse in long-term care. Nurse leadership is *the discipline and art of guiding, directing, motivating, and inspiring a group or organization toward the achievement of common goals.*[1] Another similar definition is *inspiring and catalyzing others to achieve shared goals and institutional mission in an environment where the context and meanings are evolving, thus the constant need to design new ways of achieving long-held values.*[2] In a position paper *Effective Leadership in Long Term Care*, the American College of Health Care Administrators (ACHCA) describes leadership as a position and process.[3] Although the ACHCA is an organization focused on nurse administrators,

[a] University of Arkansas for Medical Sciences, College of Nursing, 4301 West Markham Street, Slot #529, Little Rock, AR 72205, USA; [b] Ross and Carol Nese College of Nursing, Penn State University, University Park, Pennsylvania, PA 16802, USA; [c] Seton Hall University, Nutley, NJ 00710, USA
* Corresponding author.
E-mail address: harrismelodee@uams.edu

Nurs Clin N Am 57 (2022) 171–178
https://doi.org/10.1016/j.cnur.2022.02.010
0029-6465/22/© 2022 Elsevier Inc. All rights reserved.

nursing.theclinics.com

Table 1				
Registered nurse workplace comparison				
Nursing Staff	Hospital	% Employed	Nursing Home	% Employed
RN	$76,840	60%	$68,450	7%

Abbreviation: RN, registered nurse.

the position paper can apply to professional nurses in long-term care. The ACHCA identifies with the definition *the process of influencing others to understand and agree about what needs to be done and how to do it, and the process of facilitating individual and collective efforts to accomplish shared objectives.*[4] Transformational servant leadership is another approach that aligns with nurse leadership in long-term care. One definition of transformational servant leadership is *the ability to cast a collaborative moral vision while actively caring for those participating in moving the vision to reality.*[5] Visionary nurse leaders collaborate, motivate, influence, and inspire the achievement of values and goals to improve the quality of life for older adults in long-term care.

EDUCATION, LICENSURE, COMPETENCIES, AND CERTIFICATION FOR NURSE LEADERS
Education

Nurse leaders are first and foremost, registered nurses. Registered nurses may have 2 to 4 years of education and prepared at the Associate Degree in Nursing level or with a Bachelor of Science in Nursing.[6] In either educational pathway, gerontological nursing is typically integrated into the nursing curricula. According to the last survey,[7] 34% of nursing programs have stand-alone undergraduate gerontological nursing programs. Most nursing programs focus on acute care nursing. It is difficult to know if there is any preparation specific to long-term care and especially sufficient training to assume a nurse leadership role in this environment. It is more likely that professional registered nurses who choose to work in long-term care will receive much of their training on the job. The education and emphasis placed by academic institutions is reflected in the choices of professional nurses in the workforce. The pay scale is significantly lower for registered nurses in the nursing home, which may account for the alarming workforce disparities with only 7% of registered nurses choosing to work in long-term care compared with an overwhelming 60% of registered nurses who are employed in the hospital[8] (**Table 1**).

Licensure

All candidates for registered nurse licensure must pass the NCLEX-RN Examination. Candidates who successfully pass the NCLEX-RN examination may apply for licensure in the state where they intend to practice. Nurse leadership is addressed on the NCLEX blueprint. The distribution of questions relevant to nurse leadership concepts is 17% to 23% of questions related to Management of Care: Assignment, Delegation, and Supervision. The NCLEX examination tests the ability to apply the leadership concepts in nursing practice[9] (**Box 1**).

Competencies

Although underutilized, there are leadership competencies specifically for long-term care. The American Nurses Association (ANA) Leadership Advisory Council[10] (ANA, 2018) has developed ANA Leadership Competencies that are designed to apply to nurse leaders across all settings. The leadership competencies are based on the

---

Box 1
NCLEX-RN: application of leadership concepts[9]

Identify tasks for assignment or delegation based on client needs

Delegate and assign appropriate task based on client's need to personnel with competency to perform task

Assign and supervise care of client provided by others

Communicate tasks to be completed and report client concerns immediately

Organize workload to manage time effectively

Utilize the rights of if delegation

Evaluate delegated tasks to ensure correct completion of activity

Evaluate ability of staff members to perform assigned tasks considering personnel's allowable task/duties, competency, and ability to use sound judgment and decision making

Evaluate effectiveness of staff members' time management skills

Data from National Council of State Boards of Nursing, 2018.

ANA Leadership Competency Framework[10] for leading yourself, leading others, and leading the organization. The foundation for the competencies is from the *Standards of Professional Performance*.[11]

Certification as a nurse leader builds on the ANA Leadership Competency Framework and Competencies.[10] Although it is uncommon for professional registered nurses in long-term care, the American Organization of Nurse Leaders Credentialing Center[12] provides opportunities for certification as a Nurse Manager and Leader and in Executive Nursing Practice. The examinations are accredited by the National Commission for Certifying Agencies.

ORGANIZATIONS

The Geriatric Nurse Leadership Academy was funded by the Robert Wood Johnson Northwest Health Foundation and Partners Investing in Nursing.[13] The Geriatric Nurse Leadership Academy for Long-Term Care (Leadership Academy) was developed to strengthen geriatric nursing competencies and leadership skills in long-term care. The Geriatric Nurse Leadership Academy served as a platform for networking with gerontological nurse leaders and sustain the development of nurse leadership skills in geriatrics and long-term care.

The American Nurses Credentialing Center (ANCC) Pathways to Excellence in Long Term Care[14] is another model that promotes certification in leadership. For nursing homes to be eligible for this distinction, the Director of Nursing (DON) must be a baccalaureate-prepared nurse.[14] The achievements of Pathways to Excellence in Long Term Care depend on successful DONs and registered nurse leaders.

Nurses Improving Care for Healthsystem Elders (NICHE) is an organizational membership program available to facilities that provide care to older adults. The Leadership Training Program is an online education program facilitated by the NICHE team and includes asynchronous learning activities and Web-based meetings with faculty and mentors. NICHE recognizes achievements in nurse-led improvements in the care of older adults in care settings, including long-term care. The vision of NICHE is that all older adults, aged 65 years and older receive age-friendly, exemplary nursing care.[15]

CHARACTERISTICS OF NURSE LEADERS IN LONG-TERM CARE

The professional registered nurse in long-term care is described by leadership characteristics. One cross-sectional study showed 5 characteristics of nurse leaders in long-term care including experiments with new ideas, controls work closely, relies on subordinates, coaches and gives feedback, and handles conflicts in a constructive way.[16]

A model for regulation[10] for the professional registered nurse leader places self-discrimination at the top of the pyramid. Knowing one's self is an essential characteristic of the nurse leader and underlies success toward personal and professional goals and precedes understanding of institutional policies and regulation in the nursing home.

Nurse leaders in long-term care are change agents who anticipate continuously evolving policies, regulations, and priorities. Transformational leadership describes the nursing home environment. Transformational leadership involves moving the nursing home forward to forge a conceptual change in the midst of changing conditions.[2] Change is central to definitions of nursing leadership. The capacity to adapt to a changing environment is an important characteristic of a nurse leader.

Transformational leadership[1] fosters innovation. The coronavirus disease 2019 (COVID-19) crisis exemplifies innovation as an important characteristic of the nurse leader. Because of ingenuity, creativity, and the presence of nurse leaders, infection rates decreased.[17] Professional registered nurses also promote cultural change needed in nursing homes. There is over 30 years of research supports optimal outcomes for safety and quality of care. More recently, registered nurse presence predicts positive outcomes for decreasing the spread of COVID-19 in nursing homes.[17] Registered nurses in long-term care decreases hospitalizations.[18] Professional registered nurse leaders play a role in developing a culture of excellence in long-term care.[2]

ROLE OF THE NURSE LEADER AND SCOPE OF PRACTICE IN LONG-TERM CARE

Only registered nurses have the education and responsibility to assess, supervise care, and monitor the health status of nursing home residents.[19] The DON is a role of the professional registered nurse in long-term care. DONs shoulder the accountability to deliver high-quality care to nursing home residents, administrative responsibilities, management of staff, and portraying a positive image of the nursing home through partnerships.[20] The Certified Directors of Nursing examination is offered through the Certified National Association of Directors of Nursing Administration in Long Term Care.[21]

RECOMMENDATIONS

A secure and qualified workforce is needed to reform long-term care. In the current regulatory model, nurse leadership is invisible, but at the same time the first to be blamed. Expert nursing is underestimated and for the most part even discounted. The Future of Nursing Report[22] confirms and reinforces that nurse leaders will partner with other disciplines to reform health systems.

Nurse Staffing

The current regulations are outdated and can no longer be considered as evidence-based practices. The literature supports higher-than-minimum staffing levels to achieve optimal outcomes for safety and quality. It is our recommendation that Centers for Medicare and Medicaid Services (CMS) mandates adequate professional staffing in nursing homes.[19] The demand for registered nurse leadership has exceeded the supply. A mandate for nurse staffing would incentivize employers to hire registered nurses to work in long-term care. There is evidence revising regulations would result in reducing unnecessary hospitalizations, infections, falls and overall safer environment with cost saving benefits for nursing homes.[17,18]

Competencies and Certification

The current regulations for competencies are too broad. Competencies and certification should address gerontology and nurse leadership. To promote the highest standards for leadership, we are targeting recommendations for DONs.[14]

Diversity and Inclusion

Only 19.2% of the workforce includes nurses from a minority background.[23] There are disparities in access to education for minority populations, especially in rural and underserved regions where nursing homes have the greatest need for qualified expert nursing leaders. The authors recommend partnerships with academic institutions to promote recruitment of minority nurses into long-term care.[24]

Dementia Care

Owing to the growing population of older adults living with dementia, the authors recommend that schools of nursing revise curriculum to strengthen geropsychiatric nursing at the undergraduate and graduate levels. Removing scope of practice barriers for geropsychiatric nursing will provide access to expert nurses in dementia and mental health in the nursing home. Professional registered nurses lead dementia care and geropsychiatric nursing.[25]

Regulations

There are more pages of regulation associated with the nursing home than nuclear power plants.[26] The authors' recommendations point out only a few regulations that could be revised to support the nursing home environment. The changes are possible when regulation is placed into the hands of strong nursing leadership.

Excellence

To counteract a putative culture, excellence is the framework for positive reformation in long-term care. The ANCC Pathways to Excellence in Long Term Care Program[14] is one model that places a culture of excellence at the forefront and fosters nurse leadership. The Pathways for Excellence in Long Term Care[14] addresses new payment models, regulations and guidelines, caring for mental health, and staff turnover. This positive strategy relies on excellence to address professional development, shared decision making, well-being, quality, safety, and nurse leadership reflected in a positive work environment. The case for a business model is made through achieving outcomes for decreasing staff turnover, rehospitalizations, staff injury, and falls.

Restorative Justice

Nursing leadership is the key to successful outcomes in the nursing home. Under the current regulatory system, restorative justice[27] is one approach that promotes opportunities to review outcomes from a global perspective. This collaboration has been shown to be effective for nuclear power plants and nursing homes. Led by professional registered nurse leaders, input from stakeholders is solicited, and varied perspectives are considered in the transformation of health care delivery in long-term care. Restorative justice does not dismiss a negative outcome but responds with individualized regulation strategies to avoid any future negative outcomes.

In response to COVID-19, CMS[28] accelerated the amount of civil monetary penalties for nursing homes with deficiencies in infection rates. Although negligence and incompetence should be called out, there are other factors such as lack of resources and poor staffing, especially in rural and underserved nursing homes, that also contribute to infection rates for COVID-19. Increasing fines does little to decrease COVID-19. Restorative justice and responsive regulation[27,29] are a new approach for reform that can take a closer look at the vital role of nurse leadership and associated workforce needs for staffing, education, certification, resources, and reimbursement.

The authors' recommendations for placing nurse leadership on the frontlines of reform in long-term care are not new. There is 30 years of research to update and implement evidence-based practice for reform in long term. More than any other discipline, nurses know the needs of older adults living in long-term care. The proposed mandates by nursing experts in this series are designed by expert nurses to advance excellence in long-term care for older adults. As endorsed by the American College of Health Care Administrators, the best way to predict the future of long-term care is to have effective leaders create it.

CLINICS CARE POINTS

- Residents of nursing homes are at risk for poor health outcomes when professional nurse staffing standards are weak.
- Direct care workers in nursing homes need professional nurse supervision to deliver quality bedside care that promotes resident cognitive, physical, and social function.

DISCLOSURE

The authors do not have any disclosures.

REFERENCES

1. Broome ME, Marshall ES. Transformational leadership in nursing. Transformational leadership in nursing. 3rd edition. New York: Springer Publishing Company; 2021.
2. McBride A. The growth and development of nurse leaders. 2nd edition. New York: Springer Publishing Company, LLC; 2020.
3. Dana B, Olson D. Effective leadership in long-term care: the need and the opportunity. American College of Health Care Administrators; 2007. Available at: https://achca.memberclicks.net/assets/docs/ACHCA_Leadership_Need_and_Opportunity_Paper_Dana-Olson.pdf. Accessed March 25, 2022.
4. Yukl G. Leadership in organizations. 8th edition. Upper Saddle River (NJ): Prentice-Hall; 2013. Available at: http://www.mim.ac.mw/books/Leadership%20in%20Organizations%20by%20Gary%20Yukl.pdf.No1fvHJjqGHg1RgmjuyjD0oYNhx7MNeo. Accessed March 25, 2022.
5. Parolini J. Transformational servant leadership. United States: Parolini; 2012.
6. Harahan M, Stone RI, Shah P. Examining the competencies for the long-term care workforce: a status report and next steps. USA: Department of Health and Human Services; 2009. Available at: http://aspe.hhs.gov/daltcp/reports/2009/examcomp.pdf.

7. Berman A, Mezey M, Kobayashi M, et al. Gerontological nursing content in baccalaureate nursing programs: Comparison of findings from 1997 and 2003. J Prof Nurs 2005;21(5):268–75.

8. Bureau of Labor Statistics, U.S. Department of Labor, Occupational Outlook Handbook, Registered Nurses. 2021. Available at: https://www.bls.gov/ooh/healthcare/registered-nurses.htm. Accessed September 8, 2021.

9. National Council of state Boards of Nursing. 2019 NCLEX-RN test plan. Chicago: Author; 2018.

10. American Nurses Association. ANA leadership competency model 2018.. 2018. Available at: https://www.nursingworld.org/~4a0a2e/globalassets/docs/ce/177626-ana-leadership-booklet-new-final.pdf.

11. American Nurses Association. The nursing standards of practice and standards of professional performance. 3rd edition. Silver Springs (MD): ANA; 2015.

12. American Organization of Nurse Leaders. AONL credentialing center certification programs. 2018. Available at: https://www.aonl.org/initiatives/certification. Accessed March 25, 2022..

13. Culross B, Cramer ME, Terry S. Strengthening nurse leadership in long-term care: a case study. J Geriatr Med Gerontol 2018;4(3). https://doi.org/10.23937/2469-5858/1510051.

14. American Nurses Credentialing Center. Pathway to excellence in long term care: creating and sustaining a culture of excellence. 2021. Available at: https://www.nursingworld.org/organizational-programs/pathway/overview/pathway-to-excellence-in-long-term-care/. Accessed March 25, 2022.

15. Nurses improving care for Healthsystem Elders (NICHE). 2021. Available at: https://nicheprogram.org. Accessed March 25, 2022.

16. Backman A, Sjogren K, Lindkvist M, et al. Characteristics of highly rated leadership in nursing homes using item response theory. J Adv Nurs 2017;73(12): 2903–13.

17. Harrington C, Ross L, Chapman S, et al. Nurse staffing and coronavirus infections in California nursing homes. Policy Polit Nurs Pract 2020;21(3):174–86.

18. Rao A, Evans L. The role of directors of nurse in cultivating nurse empowerment. Online Ann Long Term Care 2015;23(4).

19. Kolanowski A, Horgas A, Wallhagen M, et al. A call to the CMS: Mandate adequate professional nurse staffing in nursing homes. Am J Nurs 2020; 121(3):24–7.

20. Rao A, Evans L. The role of directors of nurse in cultivating nurse empowerment. Ann Long Term Care 2015.

21. NADONALTC. Nurse leader certification prep and training. 2021. Available at: https://www.nadona.org. Accessed March 25, 2022.

22. IOM (Institute of Medicine). The future of nursing: leading change, advancing health. Washington, DC: The National Academies Press; 2011.

23. Smiley RA, Lauer P, Bienemy C, et al. The 2017 national nursing workforce survey. J Nurs Regul 2018; 9(3S). Available at: https://www.journalofnursingregulation.com/article/S2155-8256(18)30131-5/fulltext. Accessed March 25, 2022.

24. National Academies of Sciences, Engineering, and Medicine. The future of nursing 2020-2030: charting a path to achieve health equity. Washington, DC: The National Academies Press; 2021. https://doi.org/10.17226/25982.

25. Harris M, Devereaux Melillo K, Keilman L, et al. GAPNA Position Statement: supporting evidence for geropsychiatric nursing as a subspecialty of gerontological advanced practice nursing. Geriatr Nurs 2021;42(1):247–50.

26. American Medical Directors Association. White paper on the survey process. 2022. Available at: https://paltc.org/amda-white-papers-and-resolution-position-statements/white-paper-survey-process. Accessed September 24, 2021.
27. Braithwaite, John, Restorative Justice and Responsive Regulation: The Question of Evidence (September 14, 2016). RegNet Research Paper No. 2016/51 (Revised version of 2014 No. 51). Available at SSRN: Available at: https://ssrn.com/abstract=2839086. Accessed March 25, 2022.
28. CMS. Center for Clinical Standards and Quality/Quality, Safety & Oversight Group. Ref: QSO-20-31-All. 2020.
29. Spanko A. As officials mull stronger nursing home enforcement, restorative justice holds the key to true reform. Skilled Nursing Home News 2020. 2020. Available at: https://skillednursingnews.com/2020/06/as-officials-mullstronger-nursing-home-enforcement-restorative-justice-holds-key-to-true-reform/. Accessed March 25, 2022.

Multidimensional Aspects of Nurse Staffing in Nursing Homes

Christine Mueller, PhD, RN, FGSA, FAAN

KEYWORDS

• Nurse staffing • Nursing homes • Nursing practice model

KEY POINTS

- Nurse staffing in nursing homes has multiple aspects that must be considered to provide quality care for residents.
- The nurse staffing framework for nursing homes provides a comprehensive and multidimensional approach leading to the desired resident, staff, and organizational outcomes.
- The nurse staffing framework for nursing homes is congruent with the facility assessment federal requirement to assure sufficient qualified nursing staff available and to provide nursing and related services to meet the residents' needs safely and in a manner that promotes each resident's rights, physical, mental and psychosocial well-being.

For decades, serious concerns have been raised about inadequate nurse staffing in nursing homes and consequent poor quality of care. Studies on nurse staffing and quality provide strong evidence that quality of care for nursing home residents has a relationship to the amount of nursing staff effort (eg, hours per resident day), nurse staff turnover, and leadership turnover.[1–5] Among the various nurse staffing types, the evidence is the most consistent for registered nurse (RN) staffing, that is, higher quality of care is associated with higher RN staffing.[5] Given this growing body of evidence, the consistent remedy proposed is mandated nurse staffing ratios or staffing standards. However, a deeper and broader perspective of nurse staffing is needed as there are multiple aspects to nurse staffing in nursing homes that need to be considered beyond the number of nurse staff and consequently the nurse staffing strategies needed to address care quality in nursing homes.

The term "nurse staffing" is a broad term and should not be defined only as of the number of nursing staff. For example, a nursing home may have a higher than the average number of RN employed, but if the RN role is focused on administrative and management functions versus direct care for residents, the professional nursing

University of Minnesota, School of Nursing, 5-140 WDH, 308 Harvard Street, Southeast, Minneapolis, MN 55455, USA
E-mail address: cmueller@umn.edu

Nurs Clin N Am 57 (2022) 179–189
https://doi.org/10.1016/j.cnur.2022.02.001
0029-6465/22/© 2022 Elsevier Inc. All rights reserved.

care needs of the residents may not be adequately addressed or met. Recruitment and retention of nursing staff is a significant factor that can affect the needed number and type of nursing staff a nursing home has to meet the needs of residents. These examples suggest that nurse staffing has to be defined and addressed in a broader context.

Nurse staffing involves determining, allocating, and delivering nursing resources and care to residents in order to achieve the desired and required quality of care and life for residents.[6] The American Nurses Association[7] outlines a framework to guide the development, implementation, and evaluation of appropriate nurse staffing plans that is congruent with a comprehensive evidence-based framework for nurse staffing in nursing homes (**Fig. 1**).[6,8,9] The framework integrates considerations for the recruitment and retention of nursing staff.

In 2016, the Centers for Medicare and Medicaid Services issued a final rule to revise the requirements that long-term care facilities must meet to participate in the Medicare and Medicaid programs.[10] A new requirement was the completion of an annual facility assessment to assure sufficient qualified nursing staff available at all times to provide nursing and related services to meet the residents' needs safely and in a manner that promotes each resident's rights, physical, mental and psychosocial well-being. The foundation of the facility assessment is assessing the resident population, specifically taking into account the acuity or level of severity and stability of the residents' diseases, conditions, and physical, functional, and cognitive limitations. The assessment of the resident population should then drive decisions about the number and type of staff as well as the skills and competencies needed by staff to deliver care to meet the residents' needs. In addition to the residents' needs and staff competencies, the facility assessment should also address the physical environment, equipment, and services to care for the resident population as well as ethnic, cultural, and religious factors related to the care needs of the residents. **Fig. 2** illustrates how the CMS required facility assessment is consistent with the variables associated with the evidence-based framework for nurse staffing in nursing homes (resident characteristics, nursing resources, professional development, and structural support). The facility assessment does not explicitly address the nursing practice model components of the framework, specifically the organization and actual delivery of nursing care to residents. Each of the components of the framework for nurse staffing in nursing homes will be further elaborated.

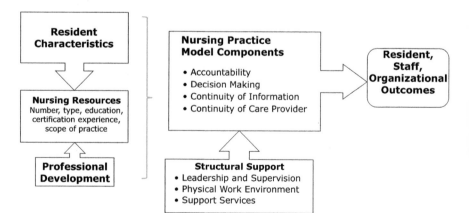

Fig. 1. Nurse staffing framework for nursing homes

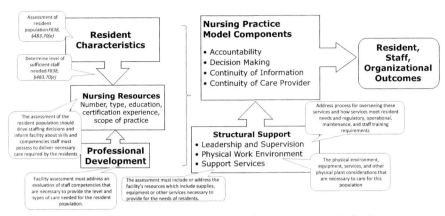

Fig. 2. Nurse staffing framework for nursing homes and CMS facility assessment requirements

Resident Needs

The needs of the residents ultimately determine the number and type of nursing staff for a nursing home. Of the over 1.2 million residents in the 15,061 nursing homes in the United States, approximately 43% are considered short-stay (length of stay <100 days) and have postacute care needs following discharge from the hospital. The other 57% are typically residing in the nursing home as their place of residence. Almost half of the nursing homes residents have Alzheimer's disease and related dementias. Nursing home residents typically have, on average, 4 activities of daily living impairments and one or more chronic health conditions. More than 60% are incontinent of bladder.[11] In general, nursing home residents need significant personal and clinical care. The stability and acuity of their clinical condition require ongoing vigilance to identify potential and actual changes in condition that can be addressed timely and proactively to avoid or prevent hospitalization and adverse outcomes.

A comprehensive nursing assessment is needed to fully address the needs of the residents. This assessment informs the development of a plan of care for each resident. Supported by federal regulations, nursing homes are required to conduct comprehensive assessments of each resident on admission and other prescribed time periods using the Resident Assessment Instrument (RAI). The RAI includes the Minimum Data Set (MDS) which is a standardized set of assessment items to inform care planning, provide nursing home level data for the assessment and reporting of quality, and determine reimbursement for care. The MDS addresses the resident's customary routines, preferences and goals of care, cognitive patterns, communication, vision and hearing, mood and behavior patterns, psychological well-being, physical functioning, continence, disease diagnosis and health conditions, dental and nutritional status, skin conditions, activity pursuits, medications, treatments and procedures and discharge planning (§483.20(b).[10] The items on the MDS trigger further assessment using 20 Care Area Assessments (CAA) such as delirium, behavioral symptoms, falls, psychotropic medication use, and pain.[12] A RN is required to conduct and coordinate the comprehensive assessments with the participation of other health professionals. The RN further coordinates the development of a comprehensive person-centered care plan that meets professional standards of quality care. The resident's goals and preferences as well as the resident's medical, physical, mental, and psychosocial needs are to be addressed in the plan of care.

Nursing Resources

The federal nursing home regulations clearly support a process to comprehensively identify the needs of the residents and a plan of care to meet those needs. The challenge is translating the residents' needs to the staff needed to meet those needs. Staffing standards for nursing home residents are, for the most part, not specific in the federal regulations. Nursing homes are required to have a licensed nurse (RN or licensed vocational/practical nurse) on staff 24 h/d 7 d/wk and 8 of those 24 hours must be staffed by an RN. The regulations provide guidelines for waivers that can be granted for the licensed nurse requirements. Otherwise, the specific regulations for nurse staffing are as follows:

"The facility must have sufficient nursing staff with the appropriate competencies and skills sets to provide nursing and related services to assure resident safety and attain or maintain the highest practicable physical, mental, and psychosocial well-being of each resident, as determined by resident assessments and individual plans of care and considering the number, acuity, and diagnoses of the facility's resident population in accordance with the facility assessment required" (§483.35) and "the facility must provide services by sufficient numbers of each of the following types of personnel (licensed nurses and other nursing personnel) on a 24-h basis to provide nursing care to all residents in accordance with resident care plans" (§483.35(a) (1).[10]

States may also have more directive staffing standards.[13] In 2001, CMS conducted a study to identify minimum staffing levels for long and short stay residents.[14] The staffing thresholds below for which residents are at risk for serious quality of care issues and above for which there were no further significant benefits related to quality if additional staffing hours per resident day are outlined in **Table 1**.

In the 20 years since those minimum staffing thresholds were identified, the nursing home population has increased in complexity and acuity. According to the most recent payroll-based journal quarterly data on nurse staffing, the average total hours per resident day (HPRD) in US nursing homes was 3.47 and RN HPRD was 0.47; significantly lower than the minimum staffing thresholds identified 20 years ago.[15]

A mechanism is needed to quantify the amount of nursing time by RNs, LP/VNs, and nursing assistants that corresponds to the needs of the residents according to their comprehensive assessment and corresponding care plan. The Resource Utilization Group Case-Mix Classification System (RUG) was developed to reimburse nursing homes based on the staffing resources needed to care for residents.[16] The RUG case-mix classification system was based on a multi-state staff time study in nursing homes to quantify the amount of nursing time, by staff type. Using the nurse staff time

Table 1 Minimum staffing levels for nursing homes		
	Short-Stay Quality Measures	Long-Stay Quality Measures
Registered Nurse Hours Per Resident Day	.55	.75
Licensed Nurse Hours Per Resident Day	1.15	1.3
Nursing Assistant Hours Per Resident Day	2.4	2.8
Total Care Hours Per Resident Day	4.1	4.85

CMS (Centers for Medicare & Medicaid Services). Appropriateness of Minimum Nurse Staffing Ratios in Nursing Homes: Report to Congress, Phase II. 2001.

and the residents' MDS data, case-mix groups were identified with associated average RN, LP/VN, and nursing assistant staff time. The staff time associated with the case-mix groups has been proposed as a means for determining nurse staffing for nursing homes.[17,18] However, the use of a case-mix or patient classification approach to quantify nurse staffing needs in nursing homes is not used by nursing homes. While nursing homes are required to conduct an annual facility assessment to determine staffing to meet the needs of the residents, there is no guidance or regulations that describe strategies or tools for quantifying staffing needs. Surveyors are provided guidance to review the facility assessment plan with a guiding question: *How did the facility determine the staffing level?*[19]

The number and type of nursing staff is only one aspect of the nursing resources needed to meet the needs of residents. The characteristics of the staff are also essential to consider, such as experience, education, competency, and scope of practice. Just as nurses need unique competencies to care for pediatric patients, so do nurses need unique competencies to care for geriatric patients. Ideally, RN hold baccalaureate degrees and have completed nursing programs that provided them with basic knowledge about the care of the geriatric patient. A variety of competencies have been identified for RN caring for older adults such as the *Recommended Baccalaureate Competencies and Curricular Guidelines for the Nursing Care of Older Adults,*[20] *Nursing Competencies for Nursing Home Culture Change,*[21,22] and *Multidisciplinary Competencies in the Care of Older Adults at the Completion of the Entry-level Health Professional Degree.*[23] The American Nurses Credential Center (ANCC) also provides certification in gerontological nursing for RN.

Competencies for nursing assistants In the care of nursing home residents are particularly important in that nursing assistants provide 80% to 90% of the direct care in nursing homes. Federal training requirements for nursing assistants are 75 initial hours with 16 clinical hours and 12 hours of annual in-service training.[10] Some states have higher required training hours. Trinkoff and colleagues[24] found that states requiring higher clinical training hours above the 16-hour minimum had a significantly lower odds of negative resident outcomes such as pain, depression and falls with injury.

The scope of practice for RNs and LP/VNs is another significant nursing resource factor to consider when determining the needed licensed nursing resources in nursing homes. Scopes of practice for RNs and LPNs are unique to each state, yet comprehensive nursing assessments, and developing, revising, and evaluating plans of care are only within the scope of practice of RNs. Given that assessment and care planning is required for every nursing home resident by federal regulations, the number of RNs should be considered particularly in that context. It is not likely that one RN staffed 7 d/wk for 8 h/d will adequately meet that federal regulation, but more importantly, address the professional nursing care needs of residents.

Recruitment and retention

Ensuring that a nursing home has the necessary qualified nursing staff to provide for the needs of the residents, recruiting and retaining nursing staff has to be a priority. Recruiting and retaining nursing staff is one of the most challenging problems in nursing homes. A recent analysis of turnover in 15,645 nursing homes using employee level data from the Payroll-Based Journal found that the average RN turnover rate was 140.7%. Average annual turnover rates for LP/VNs and NAs was 114.1% and 129.1%, respectively. Average total nursing staff turnover rates by state ranged from 39.3% to 165.1%.[25] Reasons for high turnover and low retention of nursing staff in nursing homes are related to low and noncompetitive pay and benefits, lack of respect and recognition, difficult and challenging physical work, and lack of positive relationships with supervisors. Berridge and colleagues[26] found that staff empowerment was positively associated with high retention of nursing assistants. Empowerment is further described as part of the nursing practice model.

Factors unique to the recruitment and retention of RN in nursing homes is the stigma of working in a nursing home and perception that the RN is less qualified and capable than RNs employed in hospitals. Other unique factors are the lack of a supportive professional practice environment for RNs that engages them in decision making related to their professional practice and limited support for professional development. RN' engagement in decision making regarding their work environment and resident care policies and practices, as well as having leadership in quality improvement initiatives are components of the nursing practice model that will be further elaborated with the nursing practice model components (see **Fig. 1**).

Professional Development

As previously described, nursing homes are required to provide a minimum of 12 hours of in-service training for nursing assistants on an annual basis. In addition, all nursing home direct care staff are required to have annual training on topics such as resident's rights, communication, resident abuse, neglect and exploitation, dementia care, infection control, compliance and ethics, and quality assurance and performance improvement. The development and coordination of these annual required in-service training topics most often occur through a licensed nurse that has responsibilities for staff development.

Over and above addressing the required training topics, opportunities for professional development should be identified based on the competencies needed for RNs, LP/VNs, and CNAs. Assessment skills need to be highly honed to detect the subtle changes in a resident's condition that could result in hospitalization or death. New procedures with sophisticated equipment to support the care for postacute residents need to be learned by licensed nurses. Remaining current in evidence-based practices related to the care of persons with delirium, dementia, incontinence, pressure injuries, and pain is ongoing professional development needs to ensure quality care for residents. RN, who are ultimately accountable for the care of the residents, require competency training in supervision and leadership as they oversee and direct the care provided by LP/VNs and nursing assistants.

Nursing Practice model

Once the number and type of nursing staff are determined to safely and adequately address the quality of care and life needs of the residents, the focus needs to turn to how to most effectively and efficiently organize and deliver the care. The typical approach to the organization and delivery of care used in many nursing homes is through a "task lens." Staff are assigned tasks that are congruent with their job descriptions. For example, licensed nurses administer medications and nursing assistants provide personal care for the residents such as dressing, bathing, and eating. The evidence-based nursing practice model in **Fig. 1** identifies four components that shape the approach to the organization and delivery of care through a "person-centered lens."

Accountability

The component of accountability focuses on the role of the RN who has responsibility and authority over the assessment, planning, implementation, and evaluation of nursing care for the residents. Within the RN's scope of practice, the RN also delegates, supervises, and oversees the care of residents. Mueller and colleagues[27] found that RNs and LP/VNs were used interchangeably in nursing homes. Interchangeability occurs when RNs and LP/VNs are perceived as equivalent with no acknowledgment of their differences in education and scopes of practice. Given the evidence of the association of high RN staffing and better quality care outcomes in nursing homes, the accountability component of the practice model, which takes advantage of the full scope of practice of the RN, is essential for quality of care resident outcomes.

Related to the accountability of the RN is the role of the RN in providing and promoting person-directed care in 4 areas: care role model, gerontological nurse, care partner, and teaching and mentor.[28] The *care role model* is about being a role model that supports and exemplifies person-directed care. The nurse knows the resident and is in relationship with them; this enables the nurse to effectively address their clinical needs, support their wellness, recognize their abilities, and use their strengths as assets in overcoming and addressing needs. Most importantly, the care role model for the nurse supports the person-hood of the resident and is congruent with the accountability of the RN.

The gerontological nurse role focuses on the expertise of the nurse in caring for older adults, especially those that are frail, have complex, multiple health conditions. The gerontological nurse considers the biological, social, psychological, physical, and spiritual aspects of aging in assessment, planning, implementing, and evaluating care. The gerontological nurse applies assessment and practice interventions that are evidence-based; well-grounded and staying up-to-date on gerontological nursing research and clinical practice guidelines. As a *gerontological nurse expert*, the RN would use evidence-based interventions to develop and initiate a plan of care for residents.

The RN is the clinical leader but also a *care partner* with other staff members. As the clinical expert, the RN partners with the other members of the nursing team to ensure that the clinical needs of the residents are met. And, as a care partner, the RN develops and maintains relationship and supports teamwork with other members of the nursing team to ensure a coordinated and supportive approach to the care of the residents.

Decision making

Engagement of nursing staff in making decisions about their work, their work environment, and the care of the residents/patients is essential to the organization and delivery of care as they are at the front line of care; they see and experience what can be improved and what does not work. Engagement of staff in decision making is a key component to increasing staff retention as evidenced by the use of staff empowerment strategies such as CNA involvement in care planning and day-to-day decision making.[26,29–32] An example of RN decision making (or participating in decisions about the care of residents/patients) is developing evidence-based nursing policies and procedures that will be used for the care of residents. Examples of all nursing staff decision making (or participating in the work environment decisions) is determining the supplies or equipment that will be used to ensure safe, quality resident care or making decisions about how they will do daily rounds on their unit or structure shift report. As a *mentor and teacher*, the RN continually supports learning, professional development, and coaching for the members of the nursing team—this enables staff to increase their competency in caring for residents, resulting in better outcomes, and to promote a learning community culture with the nursing staff.

Continuity of information

Continuity of information is core to the success of implementing many quality improvement initiatives such as reducing the use of antipsychotic medications or preventing hospitalizations. Continuity of information is defined as follows: adequate and relevant information about the resident/patient is available, used, and transferred among persons involved in the care of the resident/patient.[9] There are numerous strategies that can be used to ensure continuity of information. Some examples include huddles, use of SBAR, and resident rounds when doing shift reports. Strategies for how the resident's care plan is efficiently made accessible to those providing care is another example of continuity of information.

While the original component of collaboration was not validated when the nursing practice model was tested,[9] the notion of collaboration is relevant to the continuity of information. Collaboration is the extent to which nursing staff and other disciplinary staff work together to identify and meet the resident's needs. Examples include how the licensed nurses collaborate with physicians and nurse practitioners to support and coordinate the clinical needs of the residents or how the nursing assistants collaborate with the staff in the kitchen to provide meals in a timely way that also ensures the residents' food preferences are honored. As a *care partner*, the RN would ensure the nursing team members are regularly engaged in receiving and providing information about the needs and status of residents.

Continuity of care provider

Continuity of care provider is having a consistent nurse or group of nursing staff coordinating and providing care to the resident.[9] Quality nursing care is strongly supported when licensed and unlicensed nursing staff are familiar with the residents and have been able to develop relationships with them. This cannot occur if nursing staff are assigned to different residents every time they come to work. Castle[33] found that nursing homes using recommended consistent assignment guidelines had significant lower rates of turnover and absenteeism. As a *care role model*, the RN would promote continuity of care by ensuring that there are strong and sustaining relationships among residents and staff so that the residents receive individualized care and that person-directed care is supported.

The components of an NPM can be individualized to nursing homes. There is not a "one size fits all." What needs to be examined, analyzed, and evaluated in every nursing home is how the RN is accountable for addressing and meeting the professional nursing care needs of residents, how nursing staff are engaged in decision making regarding the care of residents, and how work is accomplished, how information about residents is shared, how staff are assigned to ensure continuity of care provider and the extent/degree to which there is a collaboration among other health care providers to meet the needs of the residents.

Structural Support

The facility assessment required by the CMS nursing home regulations also supports, to some extent, the structural support factors in this nursing home staffing framework (see **Fig. 2**). Leadership and supervision are essential to support staff as they deliver care. While the RN has leadership and supervision responsibilities, the director of nursing is pivotal to providing the overall leadership for the nursing department and through that leadership influences resident, staff, and organizational outcomes. Both the American Association of Directors of Nursing Services[34] and the American Organization of Nursing Leaders[35] identify leadership as a core competency for the director of nursing.

The physical work environment for the nursing staff can negatively or positively influence their ability to effectively and efficiently provide care to residents. The layout of the work area, the accessibility of supplies and linens, the location of computers for the electronic documentation of care are examples of the physical work environment. A simple scenario is whereby an RN is caring for a resident that is at the end of a hallway and receives a call back from a nurse practitioner. However, there is only one telephone at the nurse's work area and the work area is at the opposite end of a hallway. The nurse uses a lot of time going back and forth to answer phone calls, when solutions such as phones mounted in the middle of the hallways or the use of cell phones could resolve that issue and support the nurse to do his/her work more efficiently and effectively. Another significant structural support is the availability of nonnursing personnel to handle paperwork and unit administrative work (eg, faxing things to the pharmacy; ordering supplies; transcribing orders; scheduling outside appointments for residents), transporting residents, and additional staff to assist residents with eating.

Resident, Staff, and Organizational Outcomes

The nurse staffing framework for nursing homes provides a comprehensive and multidimensional approach leading to the desired resident, staff, and organizational outcomes. The components and relationships proposed in the framework will lead to better and improved quality of care and life for residents that can be evident through monitoring the CMS quality measures (eg, hospitalizations, antipsychotic medication use, falls with major injury, pressure injuries, symptoms of depression). The staffing framework is also intended to lead to positive staff outcomes such as satisfaction. Organizational outcomes can be positively impacted through a comprehensive approach to staffing such as fewer survey deficiencies and improved staff retention and lower staff turnover.

In summary, the nurse staffing framework for nursing homes is congruent with the facility assessment federal requirement. The nursing practice model components that are also included in the framework have received less attention in the context of nurse staffing, yet are essential to ensure each resident receives the care based on their comprehensive assessment and care plan. Further research is needed to test different care delivery and organization models for nursing homes that are based on the 4 nursing practice model components. Other research is needed to design and test systems that can quantify the nursing resources needed to meet the needs of the residents.

DISCLOSURE

I verify that I do not have any commercial or conflicts of interest or any funding sources.

REFERENCE

1. Castle NG. Nursing home caregiver staffing levels and quality of care: A literature review. J Appl Gerontol 2008;27(4):375–405.
2. Spilsbury K, Hewitt C, Stirk L, et al. The relationship between nurse staffing and quality of care in nursing homes: A systematic review. Int J Nurs Stud 2011;48(6): 732–50.
3. Bostik J, Rantz M, Flesner M, et al. Systematic review of studies of staffing and quality in nursing homes. JAMDA 2006;7:366–76.

4. Backhaus R, Verbeek H, Rossum E, et al. Nurse staffing impact on quality of care in nursing homes: A systematic review of longitudinal studies. JAMDA 2013;15: 383–93.

5. Dellefield M, Castle NG, McGilton K, et al. The relationship between registered nurses and nursing home quality: An integrative review (2008-2014). Nurs Econ 2015;3(2):95–108.

6. Mueller C. Nurse staffing in long-term care facilities. J Nurs Adm 2002;32(12): 640–7.

7. ANA (American Nurses Association). ANA's principles for nurse staffing. 3rd edition. Silver Springs, MD: ANA; 2020.

8. Mueller CA. framework for nurse staffing in long-term care facilities. Geriatr Nurs 2000;21(5):262–7.

9. Mueller C, Savik K. Nursing practice models in long-term care. Res Gerontological Nurs 2010;3(4):270–81.

10. CMS (Centers for Medicare and Medicaid Services). Medicare and Medicaid Programs; Reform of Requirements for Long-Term Care Facilities. Fed Regist 2016; 81(192).

11. Harris-Kojetin L, Sengupta M, Lendon JP, et al. Long-term care providers and services users in the United States, 2015–2016. National Center for Health Statistics. Vital Health Stat 2019;3(43).

12. CMS (Centers for Medicare and Medicaid Services). Long-term Care Resident Assessment Instrument 3.0 Users Manual Version 1.17.1; 2019.

13. Harrington C. Nursing home staffing standards in state statutes and regulations. 2010. Available at: https://theconsumervoice.org/uploads/files/issues/Harrington-state-staffing-table-2010.pdf. Accessed July 5, 2021.

14. CMS (Centers for Medicare & Medicaid Services). Appropriateness of Minimum Nurse Staffing Ratios in Nursing Homes: Report to Congress, Phase II. 2001. Available at: https://theconsumervoice.org/uploads/files/issues/CMS-Staffing-Study-Phase-II.pdf. Accessed May 26, 2021.

15. Long-term Care Community Coalition. Nursing home staffing 2020 Q4. Available at: https://nursinghome411.org/data/staffing/. Accessed July 7, 2021.

16. Fries B, Schneider D, Foley W, et al. Refining a case-mix measure for nursing homes: Resource Utilization Groups (RUGs-III). Med Care 1994;32(7):668–85.

17. Harrington C, Dellefield ME, Halifax E, Fleming ML M, et al. Appropriate nurse staffing levels for U.S. nursing homes. Health Serv Insights 2020;13. 1178632920934785.

18. Mueller C. The RUG-III case-mix classification system for long-term care facilities: Is it adequate for nurse staffing? J Nurs Adm 2002;30(11):535–43.

19. CMS (Centers for Medicare & Medicaid Services). State operations manual appendix PP –guidance to surveyors for long term care facilities (Rev. 11-22-17). Available at: https://www.cms.gov/Medicare/Provider-Enrollment-and-Certification/GuidanceforLawsAndRegulations/Nursing-Homes.html.

20. Hartford Geriatric Nursing Institute (HGNI) & American Association of Colleges of Nursing (AACN). Baccalaureate competencies and Curricular guidelines for the nursing care of older adults 2010.

21. Mueller C, Burger S, Rader J, et al. Nurse competencies for person directed care in nursing homes. Geriatr Nurs 2013;34(2):101–4.

22. Pioneer Network. Nurse Competencies for Nursing Home Culture Change. 2010. Available at: https://www.pioneernetwork.net/wp-content/uploads/2016/10/Nursing-Competencies-for-Culture-Change.pdf. Accessed July 7, 2021.

23. Partnership for Health in Aging. Multidisciplinary competencies in the care of older adults at the completion of the Entry-level health professional degree 2008. Available at: https://www.americangeriatrics.org/geriatrics-profession/core-competencies. Accessed July 5, 2021.

24. Trinkoff AM, Storr CL, Lerner NB, et al. CNA training requirements and resident care outcomes in nursing homes. The Gerontologist 2016;57(3):501–8.

25. Gandhi A, Yu H, Grabowski DC. High nursing staff turnover in nursing homes offers important quality information. Health Aff 2021;40(3):384–91.

26. Berridge C, Tyler DA, Miller SC. Staff empowerment practices and CNA retention: Findings from a nationally representative nursing home culture change survey. J Appl Gerontol 2018;37(4):419–34.

27. Mueller C, Duan Y, Vogelsmeier A, et al. Interchangeability of licensed nurses in nursing homes: Perspectives of directors of nursing. Nurs Outlook 2018;66(6):560–9.

28. Mueller C, Ortigara A, Misorski S. The role of the nurse in person-directed care: After 20 years of "culture change" what have we learned? Generations 2016;41:106–14.

29. Barry T, Brannon D, Mor V. Nurse aide empowerment strategies and staff stability: Effects on nursing home resident outcomes. Gerontologist 2005;45(3):309–17.

30. Cready C, Yeatts D, Gosdin M, et al. CNA empowerment: Effects on job performance and work attitudes. J Gerontol Nurs 2008;34(3):26–35.

31. Berridge C, Lima J, Schwartz M, et al. Leadership, staff empowerment, and the retention of nursing assistants: Findings from a survey of U.S. nursing homes. JAMDA 2020,21(9).124–59.

32. Hamann D. Does empowering resident families or nursing home employees in decision making improve service quality. J Appl Gerontol 2014;33(5):603–23.

33. Castle NG. Consistent assignment of nurse aides: Association with turnover and absenteeism. J Aging Soc Policy 2013;25(1):48–64.

34. AADNS (American Association of Directors of Nursing Services). DNS-CT candidate handbook. American Association of Post-acute Care Nursing; 2021.

35. AONE, AONL (American Organization of Nurse Executives, American Organization for Nursing Leadership). AONL Nurse Executive Competencies: Post-acute Care. Chicago, IL: AONE, AONL; 2015.

Age-Friendly Nursing Homes

Opportunity for Nurses to Lead

Alice Bonner, PhD, RN[a,*], Terry Fulmer, PhD, RN[b], Leslie Pelton, MPA[a],
Marina Renton, MPhil[a]

KEYWORDS

- Age-friendly • Nursing home • Leadership • Certified nursing assistant • COVID-19
- Pandemic • Huddles • Nursing home resident

KEY POINTS

- Age-Friendly Health Systems is a movement that supports comprehensive, person-centered care and support for older adults across health settings and communities.
- Nursing homes are essential to the Age-Friendly Health System movement's spread, scale, and success.
- Nursing home leaders promote staff support, team member professional development, and training as part of becoming an Age-Friendly Nursing Home.
- Age-Friendly principles are consistent with nursing home quality standards and What Matters to each older adult.

VOLUME: NURSING LEADERSHIP IN LONG TERM CARE

Introduction

Age-Friendly Health Systems (AFHS) is a movement to ensure that all care and support for and with older adults across all settings is age-friendly care. Health systems usually include multiple partner organizations; however, one type of setting that is not always engaged is the nursing home. While we will focus on Age-Friendly Nursing Homes, Age-Friendly initiatives apply to communities (including public health), universities, employers/businesses, and other organizations.[1,2] It is within the larger context of towns, cities, counties, regions, states and federal government that we consider how programs and services to support older adults can create and sustain an Age-Friendly Ecosystem, including a meaningful role for nursing homes.[3,4]

Age-Friendly care can be achieved by fully addressing its component *4 Ms.* The 4 Ms include What *M*atters, *M*edication, *M*entation and *M*obility. Age-Friendly care:

[a] Institute for Healthcare Improvement, 53 State Street, 18th Floor, Boston, MA 02109, USA;
[b] John A. Hartford Foundation, 55 East 59th Street, 16th Floor, New York, NY 10022, USA
* Corresponding author
E-mail address: abonner@ihi.org
Twitter: @TheIHI; #AgeFriendlyHealthSystems (A.B.)

Nurs Clin N Am 57 (2022) 191–206
https://doi.org/10.1016/j.cnur.2022.02.002
0029-6465/22/© 2022 Elsevier Inc. All rights reserved.

nursing.theclinics.com

- Is guided by an essential set of evidence-based practices (4 Ms, **Fig. 1**);
- Causes no harms;
- Is consistent with *What Matters* to the older adult.[5,6]

The 4 Ms framework is designed *as a set of all 4 Ms*. While health systems may initially focus on 1 or 2 of the 4 Ms to sequence becoming Age-Friendly, the team must eventually include all of the 4 Ms as a set, in workflow and care processes across departments and locations of care. Communication and public announcements regarding how and why a health system delivers Age-Friendly care is important to local communities and municipal leaders who can support and promote the value that older adults bring to their neighborhoods and communities.[7,8]

When we introduce the concept of Age-Friendly care to organizations that have traditionally focused on care and support for older adults, such as nursing homes, we often hear, "We are already doing that." We have learned that in many cases, nursing homes may be doing some 4 Ms care, some of the time, with some of the residents, and with some of the nursing home team members. But Age-Friendly care means that *all* residents receive 4 Ms care *all* of the time from *all* of the staff. That goal of 100% consistency and reliability is an essential element of Age-Friendly care.[9]

An important goal of this work is that any older adult, employee, or member of the community can articulate what is included in the 4 Ms and why the set is important. Further, the ability to articulate how the 4 Ms framework optimizes quality of life for older adults, care partners, and community members, and promotes greater joy in work for health care staff are indicators of true progress. Providing equitable, accessible Age-Friendly care and support for all older adults is a vital issue, one which requires focus and commitment.[10,11]

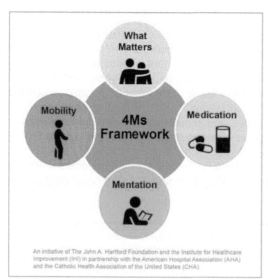

What Matters
Know and align care with each older adult's specific health outcome goals and care preferences including, but not limited to, advance care planning and goals of care, and across settings of care.

Medication
If medication is necessary, use Age-Friendly medication that does not interfere with What Matters to the older adult, Mobility, or Mentation across settings of care.

Mentation
Prevent, identify, treat, and manage dementia, depression, and delirium across settings of care.

Mobility
Ensure that older adults move safely every day in order to maintain function and do What Matters.

An initiative of The John A. Hartford Foundation and the Institute for Healthcare Improvement (IHI) in partnership with the American Hospital Association (AHA) and the Catholic Health Association of the United States (CHA).

Fig. 1. 4 Ms framework. (Source: © From Age-Friendly Health Systems an initiative of The John A. Hartford Foundation and the Institute for Healthcare Improvement (IHI) in partnership with the American Hospital Association (AHA) and the Catholic Health Association of the United States (CHA).)

DEFINITIONS AND DESCRIPTIONS
Age-Friendly

Age-Friendly care can be interpreted to mean different things depending on the context and program intent. Within the Age-Friendly Health Systems movement, Age-Friendly care refers to a practice framework in which all 4 Ms, as the essential set of evidence-based care, are practiced consistently and reliably with older adults across race and ethnicity. In an Age-Friendly nursing home, each person (clinical and nonclinical) on the team receives training and support in 4 Ms care. For example, an aide who works in nutrition services benefits from knowing how to promote a resident's mobility (eg, ability to walk to the dining room) for that person to enjoy meals in their preferred setting.

Nursing Home

The term "nursing home" generally refers to a congregate long-term care setting in which people may transition for a few days or weeks between hospital and home in the community (often referred to as a skilled nursing and rehabilitation facility or SNF), or whereby they may reside longer-term (nursing facility or NF). In many cases, nursing homes now have both SNF-certified and NF beds or rooms; therefore, they may be considered to be SNF/NFs under the code of federal regulations or CFR.[12]

The difference between an SNF and an NF is important because payment mechanisms vary depending on the care setting. SNF care is often covered by Medicare Part A or another acute/postacute care insurance benefit, whereas NF care is most often paid for either privately or under Medicaid after an individual has spent down his or her savings and assets.[13,14]

Staffing levels may also be higher in an SNF than an NF, as the clinical skills needed in an SNF may require more registered nurse (RN) and therapy coverage, additional care management, and/or social work interventions. The workflow in SNFs is more likely to have an interprofessional team dedicated to helping patients or residents meet specific goals; often those goals focus on returning to the person's home and community.[15] NF care focuses more on creating a homelike environment whereby person-centered or person-directed care drives daily routines and promotes quality of life.[16,17]

Most organizations are moving away from referring to nursing homes as "facilities," as that term emphasizes the physical building as opposed to the clinicians and other staff members who are essential to creating a positive environment for support and healing. Because the terms SNF and NF are used in regulations, we will use that language when discussing Age-Friendly care in a regulatory context.

Registered Nurses and Licensed Practical Nurses

The roles of RNs and licensed practical or vocational nurses (LPNs or LVNs) may differ in nursing homes from other settings. In nursing homes, RNs are primarily in administrative roles such as the Director of Nursing (DON) or Director of Quality and Safety and do not spend as much time with residents as the LPNs. Federal staffing regulations simply require "sufficient quality and quantity of staff" to care for residents who have been admitted to the nursing home; the Centers for Medicare and Medicaid Services (CMS) does not require minimum staffing ratios.[18]

BRIEF OVERVIEW OF AGE-FRIENDLY HEALTH SYSTEMS
History

Recent publications have outlined the history of the Age-Friendly movement.[19–21] The movement is intentionally growing to include more and more settings of care. It started with a focus on hospitals and practices, including primary care and specialty care, convenient care clinics, community health centers, and Program for All-Inclusive Care for the Elderly (PACE) programs. The movement is now expanding into nursing homes and home-based primary care in the Veterans Health Administration. In the coming months, the movement will move toward recognizing additional care at home and assisted living residences as well as specialty care including behavioral health. This sequencing of the Age-Friendly rollout by setting has been intentional, as each environment has unique characteristics that require adaptation for measuring outcomes.

Nursing homes are essential to creating a comprehensive, integrated Age-Friendly infrastructure and ecosystem. Professionals across settings can learn to use the 4 Ms framework to describe person-directed goals, capture those goals in care plans, organize and deliver care to advance those goals, and use the goals to communicate effectively with one another across care transitions.[22]

For continuity of care, we must use a cohesive and aligned system of care and terminology.[23–25] The 4 Ms can provide the framework for aligned care across settings. Without this approach, the impact of Age-Friendly care in each setting will not be fully realized.

Nursing homes are a central part of every local community—identified by the town, city, and/or county—in which they serve the needs of older adults and care partners. Leaders can champion the 4 Ms of Age-Friendly care and use the framework to drive improvements to create and implement sustainable systems in communities to support all of us as we age.

Nursing Home Measures and Outcomes

Evaluating the impact of the Age-Friendly 4 Ms framework on clinical and workforce outcomes is adapted for each setting of care. What is consistent across settings is: (1) strong recommendation to use existing measures and to stratify those by age and (2) stratification of data by race and ethnicity to ensure all four 4 Ms are being used and are having a positive, equitable impact. Nursing homes determine which measures they use, how they collect and analyze data, and how they use those data to drive change that includes how to promote resident health and well-being and how to minimize additional work for nursing home staff. Consistent ways of measuring change and improvement ensure that progress can be tracked in a meaningful way.[26,27]

A Return on Investment (ROI) calculator, business plan design, data collection templates, and other data collection methods have been developed and made publicly available.[28–31] These tools, designed for adaptation in any setting, help nursing homes build evidence for how the Age-Friendly framework improves resident clinical outcomes, supports care partners and family members, promotes more efficient and effective work practices, enhances worker job satisfaction, and reduces turnover. These resources may also be useful in conversations with administration staff who may not understand or appreciate the benefits of Age-Friendly systems and processes.[32]

In starting the Age-Friendly journey, organizations are advised to first focus on what they are already doing and the data that they are already collecting. Nursing homes that wish to receive Medicare reimbursement already submit data to CMS regularly, and clinical quality indicators may influence the amount of reimbursement. For example, each resident must have a Minimum Data Set (MDS) completed and submitted to CMS at required intervals.[33] The MDS includes detailed clinical information about each resident that guides the development of an individualized care plan. MDS is a valuable data set for following 4 Ms care.

CMS also calculates quality measures on clinical topics such as falls with injuries, functional status, pressure ulcers, and restraint use for the CMS Five Star Quality Rating System for Nursing Homes.[34] This information is available to surveyors before inspections to guide the survey team in where to focus its time and attention. CMS Five Star Quality Ratings are publicly available and designed to provide additional data for individuals to use in selecting a nursing home.[35] They are a window into evaluating Age-Friendly care.

Measuring age-friendly nursing home care

One of the fundamentals of Age-Friendly care is to focus and build on an organization's existing strengths and processes.[36] This enables each nursing home to consider how it will build sustainable systems that support older adults and are guided by What Matters to residents and ensure that the question and experience of What Matters are asked and responded to through an equity lens. Nursing homes already collect information on care processes and practices that relate to one or more of the 4 Ms. For example, virtually every nursing home has fall prevention policies and procedures that outline steps in the process to promote mobility and reduce the risk of injuries related to falls (**Box 1**).

While some or all of this data on fall prevention may be useful in implementing Mobility within the 4 Ms, it does not completely address how to promote and monitor mobility for each resident. For example, how does the nursing home team ensure that mobility is addressed in the care plan for each new resident, and for each resident every day? How does the nursing home team ensure that therapy notes and plans are read by nursing staff and that therapists are reading nurses' and primary care providers' notes as well? What strengths and improvement needs are surfaced when the data are stratified by race and ethnicity?

Changing the care plan structure and/or electronic health record (EHR) to incorporate a specific place to document each of the 4 Ms is one approach that nursing homes have taken to embed 4 Ms care into transdisciplinary work processes.[37] This must include documentation not only in the care plan that guides licensed nursing practice but also in any certified nursing assistant (CNA) documents or care cards that are used to provide an overview of each resident's care. Physicians, nurse practitioners (NPs), or physician assistants (PAs) must also be able to easily access documents and plans developed and implemented by others on the team, and there must be open lines of communication among nursing home team members, hospitals, and primary care providers.[38]

Box 1
Topics to consider in promoting mobility and preventing injuries due to falls

Screening, Assessment, and Documentation Starting on Admission

Identification of which team member (role) is responsible for each step in the process (eg, resident, care partner or family member, nurse, physical therapist, occupational therapist, primary care provider, certified nursing assistant, social worker, pharmacist, and so forth)

Potential for duplication by multiple team members and how to avoid it

Gaps and how to fill them

How and how often to report on fall prevention to the entire interprofessional team

Documentation of resident outcomes and workflow/work processes and how to update/revise processes as needed

Recent Examples of Implementation Science and Leadership – Putting the 4 Ms into Practice

2020 National Nursing Home Rapid Response Team Huddles during the COVID-19 pandemic.

The John A. Hartford Foundation (JAHF) and the Institute for Healthcare Improvement (IHI) collaborated on a 2020 initiative to support US nursing homes during the COVID-19 pandemic. The goal was to provide a daily 20-min huddle for nursing homes to share data, policy updates, and best/better practices. While the focus was largely on infection prevention and management practices, introducing the 4 Ms provided a helpful framework for leaders to guide their teams through periods of resident and staff member anxiety, depression, exhaustion, stress, and low staffing. The 4 Ms framework enabled leaders to support staff engaged in essential but challenging pandemic practices, such as limited visitation, frequent screening, deep environmental cleaning, frequent testing, donning/doffing personal protective equipment (PPE), and others.[39]

For example, promoting mobility became extremely difficult with residents being restricted to their rooms or certain areas based on infection status (cohorting). Physical and occupational therapists and others were able to share strategies to promote mobility during the pandemic. Nursing home leaders shared how the team continued to focus on What Matters and Mentation (depression, delirium, dementia) when visitation was limited, staff changes increased, and social isolation and loneliness became more prominent among residents. Reviewing the definition of delirium and how to identify residents early in the process, particularly with hypoactive delirium, was one of the curriculum topics, as well as collaboration with the pharmacist and primary care providers related to combinations of medications. This illustrates how the 4 Ms framework can be effectively implemented even during a pandemic or other public health emergency.

Age-friendly action community

Several health systems that own or are affiliated with nursing homes have also presented best/better practices during monthly Age-Friendly Action Community calls, on National Nursing Home Huddle calls, and/or through COVID-19 pandemic initiatives. Examples have been documented and published on the IHI website as case studies.[6,40]

Policy, Regulatory Intent, and Updates

There are at least 3 sets of policies and standards to consider with respect to how nursing homes operate and how they deliver quality care. First, there is the Code of Federal Regulations (CFR) specific to nursing homes that apply across all states and territories.[12] Second, there are state-level nursing home regulations.[41,42] (While states may enact regulations that are more stringent than federal regulations, they may not implement less rigorous regulations than what CMS has published.) Third, each nursing home or nursing home company may have its own policies or guidelines that are specific to the populations that it serves.

To scale and spread Age-Friendly Health Systems to all 15,600 US nursing homes, there needs to be a clear understanding of both federal and state regulations and how those may drive individual nursing home policies and procedures. For example, if Age-Friendly principles and the 4 Ms framework are not specifically identified as a set of evidence-based practices that are critical to driving improved resident and workforce outcomes, surveyors are not likely to ask about or look for Age-Friendly care during inspections. Nursing homes tend to be focused on survey results; therefore, it is critical to clearly promote Age-Friendly principles in federal and state nursing home regulations and the surveyor training process.

In addition, individual states may have regulations or payment processes that may create barriers to nursing homes implementing the 4 Ms. For example, some states still allow 3 or 4 beds per room, leading to crowded spaces that do not permit optimal mobility or equipment use by residents and staff. Most states have nursing homes that were built decades ago and are not designed to optimize Age-Friendly care.[43] While finding and retaining sufficient and qualified staff is an ongoing and serious challenge, many states have added work to prepandemic requirements, without increasing staff resources to support the delivery of quality care. In order for nursing home teams to focus on all 4 Ms, state and federal regulations need to promote systems and processes that support workflow and promote positive views of aging (finding meaning and purpose, eliminating ageism)[44] without increasing the burden on staff.

Leadership

Great leaders have the ability to identify and recruit people with leadership potential, team spirit, and open-mindedness. They also have the ability to recognize the need for change, to help organizations prepare for and manage through change, and to articulate a clear and consistent vision for that change. Leaders need vision, creativity, energy, authority, and an ability to set strategic direction.[45]

Nursing home leadership

While substantial international research has been conducted on models of nursing leadership across settings,[46,47] nursing leadership in nursing homes has not been studied as extensively.[48,49] In part, this is due to nursing faculty attitudes that do not promote careers in long-term care settings in general or in nursing homes specifically.[50] There is a perception that RNs in nursing homes are "less than" acute care RNs and primarily do paperwork. They are not seen as leaders and mentors of LPNs, CNAs, or interprofessional teams.[51] This has discouraged nursing students from considering a nursing home career; in some cases, nursing students do not even have a clinical rotation or experience in a nursing home during their nursing program. The "hidden curriculum" sends the message that a nursing home position is a last resort.

Some nursing homes no longer encourage student placements due to fear of liability or limited RN time to spend with students. As LPNs are the prominent type of nurse/ nursing role in many nursing homes, administrators and DONs often prefer to collaborate with community colleges and LPN programs rather than RN programs.

Teamwork and interprofessional practice have been integrated into the curriculum in many nursing programs, but the nursing home setting has often been left out.[52–54] In many hospitals or ambulatory care practices, newer nurses are mentored or have a senior staff nurse serve as a partner during an orientation period. However, in nursing homes, orientation is often extremely short (1 or 2 days). New nurses are often responsible for up to 30 or more residents within a very short period of time.

In addition to limited (or nonexistent) leadership training, nurses often get no instruction on how to supervise/manage other staff such as RNs, LPNs, and CNAs and limited or no instruction on the use of newer health information technology.[55] Studies have demonstrated that organizational factors may negatively influence whether or not nursing home nurses pursue continuing education.[56] In some nursing homes, there are CNAs, LPNs and RNs who have worked there for decades and have not kept pace with new care processes.

Ideally, teams would collaborate effectively and support one another.[57] However, in nursing homes, there are high rates of turnover[58,59] among leaders and direct care staff—in many cases, more than 100% per year. Therefore, building trust and working relationships among team members is a major challenge.

Leadership is part of each person's role on a nursing home team, not just something for the DON or administrator to "own." It is part of clinical and nonclinical departments and should be promoted as a key component of each person's job on the team. Leaders help team members determine when to delegate responsibility,[60] and how to balance appropriate delegation with identifying one or more team members to play the role of champion/leader on a particular project or initiative.

Strengthening nursing home leadership

Strong nursing leadership styles may have a significant impact on daily care processes and resident outcomes.[61–63] And effective nurse leadership and organizational practices can promote direct care worker retention,[64] improve clinical and organizational skills among staff,[65] and support improved resident and care partner experience of care. Nurse leaders have the capacity to be innovators, open to testing new, creative ideas and programs and promoting quality assurance performance improvement (QAPI) and related quality principles.[66]

Better ways of evaluating whether or not an individual nursing home has implemented effective leadership principles and practices are needed. This can be more comprehensively integrated into state survey processes and reflected in measures recommended through the Quality Innovation Network/Quality Improvement Organization (QIN/QIO) program.[67,68]

Nurse leaders model the behaviors and practices that they would like to see in their staff members by setting an example themselves. Strong leadership involves coaching instead of demanding or requiring certain actions. It includes generating goodwill and showing enthusiasm for stretching to reach improved outcomes as a team. Effective leaders know when to work closely with the team to fix a particular problem or breakdown in the system and when to support the team in finding solutions themselves.

Part of modeling nurse leadership involves giving credit to anyone/everyone who brings an idea forward, developing each team member, and showing that each person is equally valued. It also involves knowing when to move forward assertively with the next steps/actions and when more planning is needed. Great leaders support interprofessional practice by continually asking for input/feedback from the team and demonstrating how they use that feedback to revise workflow, practices, and to create a solid infrastructure and foundation for a sustainable system.

Nurse leaders must know each person on the team well enough to determine if/when something may be happening to negatively impact that person's work performance. In some cases, this may be work-related; in other cases, it may be a personal issue. Intervening effectively before an issue becomes a crisis is a leadership characteristic that can be learned and improved over time.

During the first year of the COVID-19 pandemic, we saw once again that staff psycho-emotional support, mental health, and well-being are vital aspects of how we can provide quality care and retain dedicated staff.[69] A strong leader must be visible on the units, attend rounds, huddles, and/or care plan meetings with teams on a regular and frequent basis, know residents well enough to participate in team decisions, and be accessible to all staff members, residents, and care partners when needed.

The role of certified nursing assistants

A critical aspect of nurse leadership in nursing homes is for directors of nursing and nurse managers to serve as role models, to demonstrate how to promote and implement person-centered care practices and effective interpersonal skills in work processes for all staff. This is particularly important in supporting CNA career development.

CNAs spend more hours per day with residents than any other nursing home team member.[70] They often know things about a resident that no one else on staff does, such as how they like their coffee, or which sweater is their favorite. They may know what time the person prefers to get up in the morning or go to sleep at night. While these preferences should be documented and shared with the interprofessional team, processes are often not in place to facilitate that communication.[71]

Nurse leaders must recognize the critical role that CNAs play in comprehensive, Age-Friendly care and must ensure that CNAs are included in team calls/meetings, huddles, rounds, and care planning.[72] It is not acceptable to say that CNAs "cannot leave their residents" or that they were asked but declined to participate. These responses indicate flaws in the system, do not reflect shared values among team members and leadership and must be addressed as part of implementing nursing home-wide person-directed care planning and quality improvement.[73]

A Plan-Do-Study-Act (PDSA) cycle or performance improvement project (PIP) that addresses how to best engage CNA participation in resident care and organizational structure, including safety culture, could contribute to higher CNA retention.[74] The improvement project could focus on 1 or 2 aspects of CNA engagement and lead to one or more improvements over time. These may be sequenced and together build momentum to begin to transform the CNA role to a more central, prominent leader driving care processes along with residents.

Another issue that has been raised by many CNAs and organizations is the lack of a career ladder/lattice in most nursing homes. Some CNAs begin their nursing home career with an ultimate goal of becoming an LPN or RN, and there are programs in several states to support this.[75,76] However, in other cases, CNAs love their job, feel a sense of dedication to individualized care and their relationships with residents, and they do not wish to become nurses. Opportunities to invite CNA participation in their own career development, without pressuring them to become nurses, should be made available across states.

CNA career development programs by organizations such as the National Association of Health Care Assistants (NAHCA), Service Employees International Union (SEIU)/1199 and other labor groups, and some by state agencies have developed apprenticeships for CNAs. These include CNA trainer roles, CNA-medication technicians, CNA leadership roles in which CNAs manage self-directed work teams, and other CNA administrative roles on the care team. Unfortunately, many of these programs were developed using grant or foundation funding and, when the funding ended, the programs did not continue. This is another major opportunity for nursing homes right now: transforming the CNA role. We must increase respect for CNA leaders inside and outside of nursing homes, and we must fully recognize the value that CNAs bring to team-based care.

Another ongoing issue has been that the wages and benefits for CNAs are below a living wage. In some states, CNAs make $8 to 9/h; the national average is about $12 to 13/h, with very limited health and other benefits in most cases.[70,77] As minimum wage and other labor laws often drive wages in each state, the lack of coordination between health and human services agencies and labor departments creates a challenge to resolving this issue at the national or state level. Stronger integration and collaboration across agencies would enhance each community's ability to find solutions. This is a public health issue.

In addition to wage issues, CNAs' weekly hours may be reduced without adequate notification, leading CNAs (many of whom are on Medicaid) to have to find other jobs to make ends meet. CNAs are most often women, racial and/or ethnic minorities, and many are single parents.[70,77] This highlights a critical disparities issue for nurse leaders: staff who are caring for the most vulnerable populations are also vulnerable, and they are often underpaid, under-recognized, and under-appreciated.

DISCUSSION
Current Challenges, Opportunities, and Next Steps

The COVID-19 pandemic has reinforced what many of us already knew: we lack a cohesive system for long-term care in the United States. The high COVID-19 case rates and death rates among nursing home residents and workers revealed once again that this is a vulnerable resident population being cared for by a vulnerable group of under-paid, under-recognized minority workers. We must scale and spread career ladders/lattices and other opportunities for CNA career development. We must also identify and promote competitive wages and benefits for nursing home nurses, leadership training for nursing home nurses, and evaluation of leadership practices through the state survey process.

Another opportunity is to change the language we use to describe aging and aging programs and services such as nursing homes. For decades we have heard or read negative descriptions of nursing homes from the media and from people in the public who say, "Whatever happens, please don't put me in a nursing home." The term "nursing home" itself has a negative connotation, one that influences policy decisions about funding and a desire to spend more state and federal revenues on home and community-based services versus institutions. Organizations such as The Frameworks Institute[78] are working to better understand and to change the negative depiction of nursing homes and other aspects of aging programs and services.

We focused a section of this article on direct care workers (CNAs); in addition, nursing homes are experiencing staff shortages related to medical directors, nurses, directors of nursing, administrators, infection preventionists, social workers, and other roles.[79,80] The nursing home care model must be based on relationships cultivated with the entire interprofessional team. We must find new ways to recruit and retain nursing home staff and leaders.

Some improvements may be accomplished through more robust integration of state and federal agencies, collaboration among Departments of Education, Labor and Workforce, Health and Human Services, and others. We must look at successful apprenticeships, orientation, and leadership programs, workforce development efforts and determine how to scale and spread initiatives that have demonstrated value. We must carefully review state and federal policies to identify and remove potential barriers and update regulations to be consistent with current practices and deliverables.

Advocacy and Action

How do we generate momentum and motivate everyone, nursing home employees and the public alike, to demand age-friendly care? We have organizations such as the American Health Care Association (AHCA), LeadingAge, AARP, and Long-Term Care Ombudsman programs to advocate for more resources for aging programs and services, for more and better oversight,[81] for changes to the nursing home model of care and reimbursement structure.

We need to engage everyone in demanding and expecting Age-Friendly care. We need to hear their voices loud and clear, and we need to find advocates for those individuals whose voices are not heard—often they are those living in nursing homes,[82] those with cognitive or mental/behavioral health conditions, and/or those with limited care partner support.

We need advocacy at the state, federal, and local levels. How does a municipal leader, who has little or no financial interest in local nursing homes, participate in conversations about nursing home transformation? We need to find models whereby this has worked and figure out how to scale and spread to other communities.

We also need advocates who deeply understand federal and state nursing homes and related regulations. If we update regulations to align with current nursing home residents and their needs, we can better deliver services to those individuals. Many in Congress and state legislatures do not understand how nursing homes operate or what the cost and reimbursement structures are; this needs urgent attention and advocacy so that appropriate resources are dedicated to support Age-Friendly nursing home care.

SUMMARY

Providing equitable, accessible, Age-Friendly care and support for and with all older adults is a vital public health issue and one which can no longer be ignored. We need to get from where we are today and where we have been to a transformational model of care and support (and a new name) for nursing homes. Nursing professionals and other long-term care leaders, public health leaders and communities are perfectly poised to accept this challenge and lead together.

CLINICS CARE POINTS

- Ask members of the interprofessional team on each floor or unit how they would structure timely, effective team meetings (huddles) and select a date to begin a small test of change

- Meet 1:1 with each certified nursing assistant (CNA) and ask them what their top 1 to 3 improvement priorities are (how to improve work-life)

- Outline how to engage team members in case reviews. Request that each team member present a case illustrating how the 4M framework was applied with a particular resident and what the outcomes were

- Include residents and (if appropriate) care partners in goal setting and care planning for each resident. Document those conversations whereby they are accessible for all relevant team members

- Use data that the nursing home is already collecting as much as possible when tracking progress on the path to Age-Friendly care.

DISCLOSURE

The authors have nothing to disclose.

REFERENCES

1. Carmody J, Black K, Bonner A, et al. Advancing Gerontological Nursing at the Intersection of Age-Friendly Communities, Health Systems, and Public Health. J Gerontol Nurs 2021;47(3):13–7.
2. Wolfe M, De Biasi A, Carmody J, et al. Expanding Public Health Practice to Address Older Adult Health and Well-being [published online ahead of print, 2020 Sep 9]. J Public Health Manag Pract 2020. https://doi.org/10.1097/PHH.0000000000001238.

3. van Hoof J, Marston HR. Age-Friendly Cities and Communities: State of the Art and Future Perspectives. Int J Environ Res Public Health 2021;18(4):1644.

4. Fulmer T, Patel P, Levy N, et al. Moving Toward a Global Age-Friendly Ecosystem. J Am Geriatr Soc 2020;68(9):1936–40.

5. Mate K, Fulmer T, Pelton L, et al. Evidence for the 4Ms: Interactions and Outcomes across the Care Continuum [published online ahead of print, 2021 Feb 8]. J Aging Health 2021. https://doi.org/10.1177/0898264321991658. 898264321991658.

6. What is an Age-Friendly Health System? Institute for Healthcare Improvement. Available at: http://www.ihi.org/Engage/Initiatives/Age-Friendly-Health-Systems/Pages/default.aspx. Accessed April 13, 2021.

7. Jeste DV, Blazer DG 2nd, Buckwalter KC, et al. Age-Friendly Communities Initiative: Public Health Approach to Promoting Successful Aging. Am J Geriatr Psychiatry 2016;24(12):1158–70.

8. DeLange Martinez P, Nakayama C, Young HM. Age-Friendly Cities During a Global Pandemic. J Gerontol Nurs 2020;46(12):7–13.

9. Age-Friendly Health Systems. Guide to using the 4Ms in the care of older adults. Boston, Massachusetts: Institute for Healthcare Improvement; 2020. p. 6. Available at: http://www.ihi.org/Engage/Initiatives/Age-Friendly-Health-Systems/Documents/IHIAgeFriendlyHealthSystems_GuidetoUsing4MsCare.pdf. Accessed April 13, 2021.

10. De Biasi A, Wolfe M, Carmody J, et al. Creating an Age-Friendly Public Health System. Innov Aging 2020;4(1):igz044.

11. Ouslander JG, Grabowski DC. COVID-19 in Nursing Homes: Calming the Perfect Storm. J Am Geriatr Soc 2020;68(10):2153–62.

12. Nursing Homes. CMS.gov. 2021. Available at: https://www.cms.gov/Medicare/Provider-Enrollment-and-Certification/GuidanceforLawsAndRegulations/Nursing-Homes. Accessed April 16, 2021.

13. Rudowitz R, Garfield R, Hinton E. 10 Things to Know About Medicaid: Setting the Facts Straight. Kaiser Family Foundation. 2019. Available at: https://www.kff.org/medicaid/issue-brief/10-things-to-know-about-medicaid-setting-the-facts-straight/. Accessed April 16, 2021.

14. Spending Down Assets to Become Medicaid Eligible for Nursing Home/Long Term Care. American Council on Aging. 2021. Available at: https://www.medicaidplanningassistance.org/medicaid-spend-down/. Accessed: April 16, 2021.

15. Vanleerberghe P, De Witte N, Claes C, et al. The quality of life of older people aging in place: a literature review. Qual Life Res 2017;26:2899–907. https://doi.org/10.1007/s11136-017-1651-0.

16. Woolcott G, Keast R, Tsasis P, et al. Reconceptualising Person-Centered Service Models as Social Ecology Networks in Supporting Integrated Care. Int J Integr Care 2019;19(2):11.

17. Lima JC, Schwartz ML, Clark MA, et al. The Changing Adoption of Culture Change Practices in U.S. Nursing Homes. Innov Aging 2020;4(3):igaa012.

18. Harrington C, Dellefield ME, Halifax E, et al. Appropriate Nurse Staffing Levels for U.S. Nursing Homes. Health Serv Insights 2020;13. https://doi.org/10.1177/1178632920934785. 1178632920934785.

19. Allen K, Ouslander JG. Age-Friendly Health Systems: Their Time Has Come. J Am Geriatr Soc 2018;66(1):19–21.

20. Mate KS, Berman A, Laderman M, et al. Creating Age-Friendly Health Systems - A vision for better care of older adults. Healthc (Amst) 2018;6(1):4–6.

21. Pettis J. Nurses leading the way to age-friendly care using the 4Ms model. Geriatr Nurs 2020;41(2):195–7.
22. Wetle TT. Age-Friendly Ecosystems: An Aspirational Goal. J Am Geriatr Soc 2020; 68(9):1929–30.
23. Ouslander JG, Reyes B, Diaz S, et al. Thirty-Day Hospital Readmissions in a Care Transitions Program for High-Risk Older Adults. J Am Geriatr Soc 2020;68(6): 1307–12.
24. Takahashi PY, Leppin AL, Hanson GJ. Hospital to Community Transitions for Older Adults: An Update for the Practicing Clinician. Mayo Clin Proc 2020; 95(10):2253–62.
25. McGilton KS, Vellani S, Babineau J, et al. Understanding transitional care programmes for older adults who experience delayed discharge: a scoping review protocol. BMJ Open 2019;9(12):e032149.
26. Coury J, Schneider JL, Rivelli JS, et al. Applying the Plan-Do-Study-Act (PDSA) approach to a large pragmatic study involving safety net clinics. BMC Health Serv Res 2017;17(1):411.
27. Curtiss FR, Fry RN, Avey SG. Framework for Pharmacy Services Quality Improvement-A Bridge to Cross the Quality Chasm. J Manag Care Spec Pharm 2020;26(7):798–816.
28. Resources to Practice Age-Friendly Care. Institute for Healthcare Improvement. Available at: http://www.ihi.org/Engage/Initiatives/Age-Friendly-Health-Systems/Pages/Resources.aspx. Accessed April 14, 2021.
29. Age-Friendly Health Systems Initiative. John A. Hartford Foundation. Available at: https://www.johnahartford.org/grants-strategy/current-strategies/age-friendly/age-friendly-health-systems-initiative. Accessed April 14, 2021.
30. Guth A, Chou J, Courtin SO, et al. An Interdisciplinary Approach to Implementing the Age-Friendly Health System 4Ms in an Ambulatory Clinical Pathway With a Focus on Medication Safety. J Gerontol Nurs 2020;46(10):7–11.
31. Tabbush V. What Age-Friendly Care Means for the Bottom Line. April 3, 2019. Available at: http://www.ihi.org/communities/blogs/what-age-friendly-care-means-for-the-bottom-line. Accessed April 14, 2021.
32. Bachynsky N. Implications for policy: The Triple Aim, Quadruple Aim, and interprofessional collaboration. Nurs Forum 2020;55(1):54–64.
33. Minimum Data Set (MDS) 3.0 for Nursing Homes and Swing Bed Providers. CMS.gov. Updated August 7, 2020. Available at: https://www.cms.gov/Medicare/Quality-Initiatives-Patient-Assessment-Instruments/NursingHomeQualityInits/NHQIMDS30. Accessed April 14, 2021.
34. Five-Star Quality Rating System. CMS.gov. October 7. 2019. Available at: https://www.cms.gov/Medicare/Provider-Enrollment-and-Certification/Certificationand Complianc/FSQRS. Accessed April 18, 2021.
35. Find & compare nursing homes, hospitals & other providers near you. Medicare.gov. Available at: https://www.medicare.gov/care-compare/?providerType=NursingHome&redirect=true. Accessed April 18, 2021.
36. Duan Y, Mueller CA, Yu F, et al. The Effects of Nursing Home Culture Change on Resident Quality of Life in U.S. Nursing Homes: An Integrative Review [published online ahead of print, 2020 Jan 22]. Res Gerontol Nurs 2020;1–15. https://doi.org/10.3928/19404921-20200115-02.
37. Bjarnadottir RI, Herzig CTA, Travers JL, et al. Implementation of Electronic Health Records in US Nursing Homes. Comput Inform Nurs 2017;35(8):417–24.

38. Adler-Milstein J, Raphael K, Bonner A, et al. Hospital adoption of electronic health record functions to support age-friendly care: results from a national survey. J Am Med Inform Assoc 2020;27(8):1206–13.
39. Xu H, Intrator O, Bowblis JR. Shortages of Staff in Nursing Homes During the COVID-19 Pandemic: What are the Driving Factors? J Am Med Dir Assoc 2020;21(10):1371–7.
40. Dawson WD, Boucher NA, Stone R, et al. COVID-19: The Time for Collaboration Between Long-Term Services and Supports, Health Care Systems, and Public Health Is Now. Milbank Q 2021. https://doi.org/10.1111/1468-0009.12500 [published online ahead of print, 2021 Feb 16].
41. Paek SC, Zhang NJ, Wan TT, et al. The Impact of State Nursing Home Staffing Standards on Nurse Staffing Levels. Med Care Res Rev 2016;73(1):41–61.
42. Chen MM, Grabowski DC. Intended and unintended consequences of minimum staffing standards for nursing homes. Health Econ 2015;24(7):822–39.
43. Zimmerman S, Dumond-Stryker C, Tandan M, et al. Nontraditional Small House Nursing Homes Have Fewer COVID-19 Cases and Deaths. J Am Med Dir Assoc 2021;22(3):489–93.
44. Colenda CC, Reynolds CF, Applegate WB, et al. COVID-19 Pandemic and Ageism: A Call for Humanitarian Care. J Am Med Dir Assoc 2020;21(8):1005–6.
45. McKinney SH, Corazzini K, Anderson RA, et al. Nursing home director of nursing leadership style and director of nursing-sensitive survey deficiencies. Health Care Manage Rev 2016;41(3):224–32.
46. Marcellus L, Duncan S, MacKinnon K, et al. The Role of Education in Developing Leadership in Nurses. Nurs Leadersh (Tor Ont) 2018;31(4):26–35.
47. Spetz J, Stone RI, Chapman SA, et al. Home And Community-Based Workforce For Patients With Serious Illness Requires Support To Meet Growing Needs. Health Aff (Millwood) 2019;38(6):902–9.
48. Wiig S, Ree E, Johannessen T, et al. Improving quality and safety in nursing homes and home care: the study protocol of a mixed-methods research design to implement a leadership intervention. BMJ Open 2018;8(3):e020933. https://doi.org/10.1136/bmjopen-2017-020933.
49. Zonneveld N, Pittens C, Minkman M. Appropriate leadership in nursing home care: a narrative review. Leadersh Health Serv (Bradf Engl 2021. https://doi.org/10.1108/LHS-04-2020-0012. ahead-of-print(ahead-of-print):.
50. Haun CN, Mahafza ZB, Cook CL, et al. A Study Examining the Influence of Proximity to Nurse Education Resources on Quality of Care Outcomes in Nursing Homes. Inquiry 2018;55. https://doi.org/10.1177/0046958018787694. 46958018787694.
51. van Stenis AR, van Wingerden J, Kolkhuis Tanke I. The Changing Role of Health Care Professionals in Nursing Homes: A Systematic Literature Review of a Decade of Change. Front Psychol 2017;8:2008. https://doi.org/10.3389/fpsyg.2017.02008.
52. Ginsburg L, Easterbrook A, Berta W, et al. Implementing Frontline Worker-Led Quality Improvement in Nursing Homes: Getting to "How. Jt Comm J Qual Patient Saf 2018;44(9):526–35.
53. Siegel EO, Young HM, Zysberg L, et al. Securing and Managing Nursing Home Resources: Director of Nursing Tactics. Gerontologist 2015;55(5):748–59.
54. Chisholm L, Zhang NJ, Hyer K, et al. Culture Change in Nursing Homes: What Is the Role of Nursing Home Resources? Inquiry 2018;55. 46958018787043.
55. Ko M, Wagner L, Spetz J. Nursing Home Implementation of Health Information Technology: Review of the Literature Finds Inadequate Investment in Preparation,

Infrastructure, and Training. Inquiry 2018;55. https://doi.org/10.1177/0046958018778902. 46958018778902.

56. Dyck MJ, Kim MJ. Continuing Education Preferences, Facilitators, and Barriers for Nursing Home Nurses. J Contin Educ Nurs 2018;49(1):26–33.

57. Sullivan JL, Weinburg DB, Gidmark S, et al. Collaborative capacity and patient-centered care in the Veterans' Health Administration Community Living Centers. Int J Care Coord 2019;22(2):90–9.

58. Berridge C, Lima J, Schwartz M, et al. Leadership, Staff Empowerment, and the Retention of Nursing Assistants: Findings From a Survey of U.S. Nursing Homes. J Am Med Dir Assoc 2020;21(9):1254–9.e2.

59. Gandhi A, Yu H, Grabowski DC. High Nursing Staff Turnover In Nursing Homes Offers Important Quality Information. Health Aff (Millwood) 2021;40(3):384–91.

60. Corazzini KN, Anderson RA, Rapp CG, et al. Delegation in Long-term Care: Scope of practice or job description? Online J Issues Nurs 2010;15(2). https://doi.org/10.3912/OJIN.Vol15No02Man04. Manuscript 4.

61. Shin JH. Nursing Staff Characteristics on Resident Outcomes in Nursing Homes. J Nurs Res 2019;27(1):1–9.

62. Boamah S. Linking Nurses' Clinical Leadership to Patient Care Quality: The Role of Transformational Leadership and Workplace Empowerment. Can J Nurs Res 2018;50(1):9–19.

63. Kiwanuka F, Nanyonga RC, Sak-Dankosky N, et al. Nursing leadership styles and their impact on intensive care unit quality measures: An integrative review. J Nurs Manag 2021;29(2):133–42.

64. Kennedy KA, Applebaum R, Bowblis JR, et al. Organizational Factors Associated with Retention of Direct Care Workers: A Comparison of Nursing Homes and Assisted Living Facilities. Gerontologist 2020;gnaa130. https://doi.org/10.1093/geront/gnaa130 [published online ahead of print, 2020 Sep 14].

65. Vogelsmeier A, Anderson RA, Anbari A, et al. A qualitative study describing nursing home nurses sensemaking to detect medication order discrepancies. BMC Health Serv Res 2017;17(1):531. https://doi.org/10.1186/s12913-017-2495-6.

66. Williams KN, Perkhounkova Y, Bossen A, et al. Nursing Home Staff Intentions for Learned Communication Skills: Knowledge to Practice. J Gerontol Nurs 2016;42(3):26–34.

67. QIN-QIOs About. Quality Improvement Organizations. Available at: https://www.qioprogram.org/about/why-cms-has-qios. Accessed April 18, 2021.

68. Quality Improvement Organizations. CMS.gov. Updated February 11, 2020. Available at: https://www.cms.gov/Medicare/Quality-Initiatives-Patient-Assessment-Instruments/QualityImprovementOrgs. Accessed April 18, 2021.

69. White EM, Wetle TF, Reddy A, et al. Front-line Nursing Home Staff Experiences During the COVID-19 Pandemic [published correction appears in J Am Med Dir Assoc. 2021 Mar 27. J Am Med Dir Assoc 2021;22(1):199–203.

70. Campbell S, Del Rio Draka A, Espinoza R, et al. Caring for the Future: The Power and Potential of America's Direct Care Workforce. New York: PHI. 2021. Available at: https://phinational.org/resource/caring-for-the-future-the-power-and-potential-of-americas-direct-care-workforce/#:~:text='Caring%20for%20the%20Future'%20describes,the%20long%2Dterm%20care%20sector.

71. Kolanowski A, Van Haitsma K, Penrod J, et al. Wish we would have known that!" Communication Breakdown Impedes Person-Centered Care. Gerontologist 2015;55(Suppl 1):S50–60.

72. Eaton J, Cloyes K, Paulsen B, et al. Certified nursing assistants as agents of creative caregiving in long-term care. Int J Old People Nurs 2020;15(1):e12280.
73. Scales K, Lepore M, Anderson RA, et al. Person-Directed Care Planning in Nursing Homes: Resident, Family, and Staff Perspectives. J Appl Gerontol 2019;38(2):183–206.
74. Temkin-Greener H, Cen X, Li Y. Nursing Home Staff Turnover and Perceived Patient Safety Culture: Results from a National Survey. Gerontologist 2020;60(7): 1303–11.
75. CNA to LPN Programs. Practicalnursing.org. 2020. Available at: https://www. practicalnursing.org/cna-lpn-programs. Accessed April 21, 2021.
76. CNA to LPN Programs. Accredited Schools Online. Published April 16, 2021. Available at: https://www.accreditedschoolsonline.org/practical-nursing/cna-to-lpn-programs/. Accessed April 21, 2021.
77. Weller C, Almeida B, Cohen M, et al. Making Care Work Pay: How Paying At Least a Living Wage to Direct Care Workers Could Benefit Care Recipients, Workers, and Communities. Washington, DC: LeadingAge. 2020. Available at: https:// leadingage.org/sites/default/files/Making%20Care%20Work%20Pay%20Report. pdf. Accessed April 21, 2021.
78. Changing the Conversation on Social Issues. FrameWorks. Available at: https:// www.frameworksinstitute.org/. Accessed April 18, 2021.
79. Stone PW, Agarwal M, Pogorzelska-Maziarz M. Infection preventionist staffing in nursing homes. Am J Infect Control 2020;48(3):330–2.
80. Banaszak-Holl J, Intrator O, Li J, et al. The Impact of Chain Standardization on Nursing Home Staffing. Med Care 2018;56(12):994–1000.
81. Silver-Greenberg J, Gebeloff R. Maggots, Rape and Yet Five Stars: How U.S. Ratings of Nursing Homes Mislead the Public. The New York Times. March 13. 2021. Available at: https://www.nytimes.com/2021/03/13/business/nursing-homes-ratings-medicare-covid.html. Accessed April 18, 2021.
82. Shaw PA. Nursing Home Residents: Age-Friendly Communities. J Gerontological Social Work 2018;61(1):11–5.

Essential Reform in Long-Term Care

Tara A. Cortes, PhD, RN, FAAN, FGSA

KEYWORDS

• Long-term care • Leadership • Workforce • Payment

KEY POINTS

- State and federal policies for long-term care must readjust the ratio of dollars that go to profit and those that go to direct patient care.
- Reform must focus on ensuring that appropriate financial support is provided for residents in long-term care.
- With appropriate financing, minimum hours of nursing care, including a percentage of RN time, must be mandated.
- Education of nurses and direct caregivers must sufficiently prepare them to understand the multi-dimensional processes of aging and to provide age-sensitive support and care across the health care continuum.

INTRODUCTION

Our nation's 15,000 nursing homes became "ground zero" in the early days of the COVID-19 pandemic accounting for nearly 5% of all cases and nearly 40% of deaths attributed to the pandemic.[1] The virulence of COVID-19 coupled with the current state of nursing homes created the perfect storm that led to so many deaths. While the vast majority of nursing staff strived to provide the best possible care, we were witness to the impact of the shocking lack of resources and reporting that severely hampered the ability to pivot from everyday care to effective infection prevention and crisis management. The pandemic put a spotlight on the historical neglect of long-term care. Nursing homes have been marginalized, even siloed, and denied a seat at the health care table for policy and reimbursement issues.

Although residential long-term care is historically thought of as being simply custodial, the care needed in these settings is actually some of the most complex care delivered across the health care continuum. Most residents have multiple chronic diseases and very often have dementia as well. There are no protocols to prescribe care because each individual has different multiple conditions. With the increase in the

Hartford Institute for Geriatric Nursing at NYU Rory Meyers College of Nursing, 433 First Avenue Room 502, New York, NY 10010, USA
E-mail address: tc13@nyu.edu

Nurs Clin N Am 57 (2022) 207–215
https://doi.org/10.1016/j.cnur.2022.02.003
0029-6465/22/© 2022 Elsevier Inc. All rights reserved.
nursing.theclinics.com

number of people living to 85 and beyond, and the increase in complexity of those living in residential long-term care, the need for quality nursing homes—nursing homes that provide the right care at the right time by the right staff—is more acute than ever. To provide this kind of care requires leadership that understands how policy decisions made at the federal and state level have impacted the nursing homes over the years, envisions and advocates for policies that will serve our growing older population in the decades to come, and assumes responsibility for leading the industry in providing cost-effective and person-centered quality care.

Government regulation has been the method used to ensure quality care in nursing homes. The Nursing Home Reform Act was passed as part of the Omnibus Reconciliation Act of 1987 (OBRA'87).[2] It requires nursing homes participating in Medicare and Medicaid to be aligned with specific quality "rules of care." These "rules" focus on quality as well as the residents' rights and person-centered care. Embedded in the Affordable Care Act (2010) are regulations to ensure transparency and accountability in long-term care and prevent resident abuse. However, the way for which the United States regulates and pays for nursing home care has made the actual implementation of any regulations nearly impossible and this was made highly visible during COVID-19. Furthermore, regulations are largely state-driven and vary greatly from state to state. There has never been a system to use evidence as a predictor of quality to determine compliance with the "rules of care." Oversight is usually punitive resulting in fines, probation, or even closure and any remediation comes at what is often a substantial financial burden to any nursing home often requiring the engagement of outside consultants for which the nursing home absorbs the bill.

Many of the issues contributing to this perfect storm are long-standing and will necessitate both immediate response and a long-term strategy. It is time to stop blaming and look for lessons learned from the devasting loss in the wake of COVID-19. Initial responses during the pandemic included an emphasis on infection control infrastructure in long-term care and crisis management. Educational programs for all levels of nursing home staff on these issues are abundant. Nursing homes used travel nurses and agency nurses to increase needed professional staffing. Visits from outsiders were stopped and regular testing for staff and residents was made available. Many states stepped up their surveillance of infection control practices along with the fines for noncompliance. The Trump administration established a commission to make recommendations to improve the quality and safety of care in nursing homes. These were just some of the immediate responses to an overwhelming tragedy—the avoidable death of more than 40,000 residents in congregate living. However, quick fixes and reports that have no resources to enable the implementation of recommendations will only go so far. Unless we address the long-term strategies of payment reform for nursing homes which is necessary for the development of strong leadership and an appropriate workforce to navigate this industry into the future, we will leave a gap in care for those older adults who will need institutional care.

PAYMENT REFORM

One of the first issues to be addressed is for nursing homes to have adequate funding to implement evidence-based quality care for this complex population. It is essential that providers of long-term care services are at the table as full partners with hospitals when informing policy decisions. There should be a partnership formed between these 2 entities to ensure the collaboration and coordination of care as well as equitable distribution of dollars. Our society has long been hospital-centric with community-based or long-term care a second thought. During the early days of the pandemic, hospitals received the lion's share of personal protective equipment (PPE) while nursing home administrators went anywhere they could to find whatever medical supplies were needed to protect their staff. In the meantime, staff often had to use garbage bags as gowns and handkerchiefs as masks. When the CARES Act was passed in July it allocated $175B for hospitals and just $4.9 B for nursing homes affected by COVID-19.[3]

The primary payer for nursing home care is Medicaid and the payment amount varies from state to state. Unlike Medicare which adjusts rates according to the cost of care, Medicaid reimbursement is determined by state legislators and allocated annually in state budgets. Historically Medicaid has not paid nursing homes for the full cost of care and several states have not increased payments for more than 10 years despite cost-of-living changes. Notably, one state (New York) received CMS approval to decrease nursing home rates in 2020.[4] Nursing homes have been able to offset the insufficient Medicaid payment by providing short-term rehabilitation and postacute care to people who are Medicare eligible. In addition, some nursing homes have patients who pay out-of-pocket for their care which serves as another mechanism to balance their budget. However, COVID-19 decreased these revenue pipelines. Nursing homes across the country are seeing their census drop by 20% or more resulting in even less reimbursement. The decrease in elective surgeries during the pandemic reduced the number of Medicare admissions for short-term stay and today, because of the well-publicized impact of COVID-19 on nursing homes, many people are electing to go home for care after hospitalization. In addition, people are looking for alternatives to nursing home care when considering the care needed for an aging parent or spouse. And, those nursing homes which serve low-income populations in traditionally medically underserved areas have fewer opportunities to collect from Medicare or private pay and struggle even more now to continue existence. This financial impact is forcing many nursing homes, particularly those with a large number of Medicaid beneficiaries to eliminate staff, decrease beds, or even close or sell to the for-profit sector of long-term care.

Changes must be made to the financial model that has been used to pay for long-term care in this country for decades. Nursing homes receive billions of dollars each year in federal funding from Medicare and Medicaid. There needs to be accountability and transparency by nursing homes on how their revenue is used. Nursing homes are able to spend their money as they want to with no required reporting on how it was spent or on profits made. Some nursing homes have multiple entities as part of their own organization such as a physical therapy "company" with whom they contract to pay themselves back for services billed to insurance. The majority of nursing homes in this country are for profit, often in chains or corporations, and even bought as investments for venture capitalists. CMS needs to mandate audits to determine how nursing homes spend their money. These should be conducted by independent auditors and evaluated by independent contractors. Furthermore, a medical loss ratio must be established that would require a designated amount of reimbursement to be spent on the care of residents and limit the amount of the reimbursement that could be spent on administrative and management fees and profits. Some states are considering this in their 2021 legislative agenda.

A simple adjustment to the model is to ensure that payment rates to nursing homes are adjusted yearly as are Medicare rates and correspond to the cost delivery of evidence-based quality care as determined by appropriate measurements reflective of person-centered care which incorporates the wishes of the resident and of care that delivers age-sensitive outcomes. Another adjustment is to implement a pay-for-performance approach that is becoming common in other parts of the health care system. There is some limited reimbursement provided for certain factors that CMS deems related to quality, but the metrics look at specific criteria such as pressure ulcer incidence or the number of falls, but they do not measure the resident's quality of life or the degree of care planning around "what matters" to the resident. As Medicaid dollars are provided to states by the federal government, it may require more federal dollars to be distributed. However, recognizing that there is a finite amount of dollars available for any government program it is necessary to explore how to pay for any new financial model. There needs to be reform in the structure of the Medicare and Medicaid program which might require an additional Medicare tax such as a Part E and as well as more comprehensive coordination of Medicare and Medicaid benefits. There may need to be a systematic redistribution of how dollars are spent in long-term care. Payment reform in long-term care is essential if there is to be an adequate workforce prepared to meet the complex needs of our aging population.

WORKFORCE

The essential workforce in long-term care is comprised of nurses and direct caregivers. The capacity of this workforce to deliver person-centered, quality, and cost-effective care is very dependent on staffing patterns, education of that staff, both preparatory education and continuing education, and leadership. None of this, however, has ever been considered in setting policy. In fact, CMS requires only one RN for 8 h/d in a nursing home. The other 16 hours can be covered by a licensed practical nurse with less than 1 year of technical education while an RN has a college degree. The lack of adequate funding over several decades has led to the "perfect storm" we witnessed in long-term care when COVID-19 began ravaging nursing homes.

There is a wide consensus that at least 4.1 hours of care per resident by direct caregivers and nurses are necessary to avoid systematic poor care.[5] Studies also demonstrated that nursing homes with more professional nurses have fewer COVID-19 infections and fewer fatalities.[6] Considerable research has shown there must be a staff with an appropriate number of professionals and direct caregivers to provide quality care to the increasingly older and more complex population in long-term care as well as navigate through any crisis such as a pandemic.

Strong nursing leadership driving evidence-based practice improves quality and cost-effective. Several national reports have called for a strong registered nurse (RN) presence in long-term care as a critical solution to increase quality while decreasing cost to the overall system. A study conducted by the Center for Medicare and Medicaid Services (CMS) found that nursing homes with a greater RN staff number had significantly fewer hospital readmissions.[7] Another study conducted following the pandemic on all 215 nursing homes in Connecticut found that those with higher RN staffing and quality ratings better controlled the spread of the novel coronavirus and had a lower number of deaths.[8] None of this evidence, however, has ever been considered in setting policy. In fact, CMS requires only one RN for 8 h/d in a nursing home. There is no federal standard set for minimum staffing and although some states have established a minimum, that minimum is less than 4.1 hours and does not take into consideration the rising acuity and complexity of the residents today. Furthermore, nursing homes are incentivized to keep staffing numbers as low as possible because personnel costs are the main driver of expenditures. This is particularly important in the for-profit nursing homes which comprise around 70% of the industry.[9]

A Senate bill (S2943) to set a minimum staffing standard was introduced to the 116th Congress in 2019 but did not receive a single vote.[9] With COVID-19 and the tragic vulnerability to death in nursing homes has created the impetus for similar bills to be introduced to the 117th Congress. The Quality Care for Nursing Home Residents and Workers During COVID-19 and Beyond Act (H.R.598) was introduced in the House by Representative Schakowsky on 2/02/21 and The Quality Care for Nursing Home Residents Act was introduced in the Senate (S315) by Senators Blumenthal and Booker on 02/12/21.[10,11] These bills propose a federally mandated staffing minimum at 4.1 hours of nursing care per resident day with at least 0.75 hours by a RN, 0.54 hours by a licensed practical nurse and 2.81 hours by a certified nursing assistant. The passage of this bill could be transformational for long-term care, but along with minimum staffing, there will be the need for the appropriate number of staff with the right preparation to provide this care. Quality care will also require the right leadership in long-term care to recruit, support, and retain that staff.

Recruitment and retention of both professional nurses and nursing assistants have been a challenge in the long-term care industry for years and COVID-19 exacerbated turnover as staff were out sick with the virus and others fled the workplace in fear of getting sick and infecting those with whom they lived. There are many reasons, personal and professional, why people leave jobs, but job market research has shown that most often turnover is related to compensation and benefits, education to do the required work, in this case, to work with a very complex population, and leadership to foster an environment of respect and professional growth.

Historically, compensation and benefits in nursing homes have been inferior when compared with hospitals. The median salary for RNs in long-term care is $29.29/h with a high range of $36/h, while nurses in hospitals have a median salary of $32.10 with a high range of $44/h[12] Most hospitals offer tuition aid for nurses to RNs to complete the bachelor's or master's degree in nursing while few nursing homes provide that benefit.

Certified nursing assistants in nursing homes across the US have a median annual income of $28,500 with a median hourly income of $12.93 which is 13% less than the national hourly wage.[13,14] These direct care workers who are often the eyes and ears of the residents, are vastly undervalued and they are often forced to work 1 or 2 other jobs just to make a living wage. Unless competitive and livable wages are provided to the long-term care workforce recruitment and retention will continue to be a challenge.

Educational preparation of the workforce for long-term care has never been emphasized for nurses or for nursing assistants and with the increasing complexity of caring for the aging population, preparation of the workforce is more important than ever. Nursing education emphasizes acute care of the hospitalized patient once again reflecting the hospital-centric, disease-focused paradigm of health care in this country. Very often, the first clinical experience nursing students have is in a nursing home, presumably to learn how to give bed baths and take vital signs. These students are put into an environment with people who have multiple chronic diseases and dementia-specific behaviors. Students are not prepared to interact with people with dementia at this point of their education, with the result that they are afraid, feel inadequate and never want to go into a nursing home again. These experiences only reinforce negative stereotypes on aging such as frail, feeble, and dependent and do not provide insights into the many dimensions of aging which include the richness of wisdom and experience older people can share with younger generations. Nursing students should have opportunities to work with older adults in diversified settings to understand the wide spectrum of aging and health. Experience in nursing homes should be built into the curriculum when students have an understanding of chronic diseases, the behavioral and physical manifestations, and the impact of social determinants of health on the life experiences of older adults. The ability of a student to assess and develop a person-centered plan of care incorporating the individuality of what matters to that resident requires a high level of evidence-based practice and a good sense of self-confidence.

Nursing assistants (NAs) need to have appropriate education in providing care to the complex population in nursing homes. The federally mandated minimum training of 75 hours to sit for the certification examination as a nursing assistant was established in 1987. There has been no change to these minimum hours over the years despite the increasing complexity of the care needed for nursing home residents. Each year there are a certain number of hours, usually 12 to 16 hours, determined by individual states for continuing education. This education is not nearly enough to provide NAs with the confidence they need to interact with residents who have multiple chronic conditions, dementia, and often superimposed delirium. These NAs who provide most of the care to residents in long-term care need to be able to assess changes in behavior, recognize signs of failure and know what it means to provide palliative care. It is very difficult to be an engaged, confident, and satisfied team member with this minimum level of education and preparation.

LEADERSHIP

The culture of any organization is framed by a set of values that are driven throughout the organization by leadership. This culture impacts staff satisfaction and ultimately resident satisfaction. Leadership is the lynchpin between the culture of the organization and high-quality person-centered care by a committed staff. Yet, nursing homes are led by administrators who may or may not have even a bachelor's degree as there is no federal standard for the education or skills necessary to being a nursing home administrator. The Nursing Home Reform Act passed by Congress in 1987 required the Secretary of Health and Human Services to establish federal standards to regulate administrator education and licensing. Instead of establishing one overall directive, the agency delegated authority to individual states to set educational, testing, and continuing education requirements overseen by the appropriate health agency of each state. Collaboration among these state agencies led to the development of a national examination under the authority of the National Association of Long-Term Administrator Boards (NAB).[15] Although nursing home administrators do have to pass this national licensing examination, \standards vary from state to state so not all states require an additional state-level examination.

And as there is no federal standard for the education of nursing home administrators, the level of education required has much variability. While most states require a minimum of a bachelor's degree to qualify for a nursing home administrator license, some require only an associate degree and some require a master's degree in public health, nursing, long-term care administration, health services administration, or business administration.[16]

Many nursing homes use RNs as directors of nursing or as administrators. More than two-thirds of the RNs hired into nursing homes have only a 2-year Associate Degree in Nursing which prepares them as bedside nurses but includes almost no education on leadership.[17] The lack of a standard preparation of leaders in long-term care contributes to the continuation of top–down management reminiscent of the last century model of leadership. We need to develop leaders and standardize qualifications for leadership positions in long-term care that can drive a person-centered culture for residents and staff that supports decentralized decision making, collaboration and teamwork, continuous quality improvement, and a focus on quality-of-life and "what matters" for each unique resident.

To drive this type of culture, leaders need to foster leadership at every level of the organization and recognize the importance of different skill sets that people bring to organizational systems. By encouraging all employees to be proactive and have a voice in decision-making creates a culture of strength at every level. It allows the direct caregivers to lead resident care and "partner" with the residents and/or their families to share decisions in planning person-centered care. Leaders need to be prepared to share their authority and recognize that their strength comes from the people in the organization who are doing the work of the mission. It requires the leader to be confident and understand that power and authority do not come from the title but come from building respect among the team who want to help achieve the leader's goals.

A confident and prepared leader embraces the concept of "servant leadership" for which the leader helps people gain confidence and competence so they can manage their own behavior in as many aspects of their job as possible and become autonomous.[18] This leader understands the importance of shared governance which promotes shared decision-making and gives everyone a voice in their work It brings together nurses, certified nursing assistants and other direct care providers as well as residents to provide input into their environment. It promotes a safe environment in which all levels of employees feel confident, knows that they can express their ideas, get honest feedback, and are committed to organizational values. It promotes a culture that is focused on intrinsic values, not extrinsic values. Employees in this culture value organizational-wide leadership, the mission, and the satisfaction of the people they serve, and value less their pay, bonuses, and material rewards.

Some studies indicate that addressing the need for strong leadership and continued leadership development in long-term care settings is a critical factor that can improve staff recruitment and retention, improve staff satisfaction, and increase the quality of care.[17] Recruitment and retention are higher in organizations in which well-prepared leaders demonstrate respect, act with integrity and lead by influence. Respect means that each employee is acknowledged for their potential and given permission to do their best work. Integrity is demonstrated by being honest and open when communicating with others and holding yourself accountable while owning up to mistakes or shortcomings. A leader can influence through providing good communication, listening to others, and not reverting to coercion.

SUMMARY

Legislation and policy need to drive reform in long-term care. COVID-19 and the number of deaths that came in its wake was the watershed event that made public the inadequacies of an industry in crisis, yet an industry in which millions of people entrust their loved ones. The Nursing Home Reform Act of 1987 has never fulfilled its potential of advancing the quality and standards of long-term care. Instead, nursing homes have become largely proprietary, and as businesses, they calculate their services toward the profitability goals and not to the benefit of residents. First, state and federal policies for long-term care must readjust the ratio of dollars that go to profit and those that go to direct patient care.

Second, reform must focus on ensuring that appropriate financial support is provided for residents in long-term care. The prospective payment system allowed nursing homes to retain the difference between the rate and what they actually spend. However, as states control that rate, payment fluctuates with state priorities, and long-term care never seems to be state budgets' priority. Most often, this rate has not changed sufficiently over the years to keep up inflation and consequently direct services to residents have been reduced.

Third, with appropriate financing, minimum hours of nursing care, including a percentage of RN time, must be mandated. Although residents in long-term care have become more complex as the mean age of the residents' increases, staffing has remained the same or, in many cases, has decreased both in the number of RNs as well as certified nursing assistants, often to address budget shortfalls, but also due to recruitment and retention issues.

Fourth, education of nurses and direct caregivers must sufficiently prepare them to understand the multi-dimensional processes of aging and to provide age-sensitive support and care across the health care continuum. Curricula preparing professional nurses must provide appropriate educational opportunities that encompass the care of older adults whether they are in the hospital, the community, or in long-term care. Direct caregivers must have adequate training to provide the right care at the right time and promote person-centered care.

And finally, the importance of well-prepared leadership and its correlation to recruitment and retention of staff, as well as quality of person-centered care must be recognized. Federal policy needs to standardize the required education and competency for leadership in long-term care.

With the impetus of increased public awareness about the challenges of providing long-term care in this country, there is additional money and resources being directed to home and community-based services. While resources to allow people to age in place are necessary, the need for residential long-term care will not disappear. We need to ensure that our long-term care facilities have an adequate workforce with strong leadership and appropriate financial support to provide the appropriate care to people who need to have that level of skilled nursing.

DISCLOSURE

The author has nothing to disclose.

REFERENCES

1. The New York Times, Nearly one-third of U.S. Coronavirus deaths are linked to nursing homes. The New York Times. Available at: https://www.nytimes.com/interactive/2020/us/coronavirus-nursing-homes.html. Accessed 2020.
2. Israelsen-Hartley S. Will long-term care be the same after COVID-19? Deseret News. Available at: https://www.deseret.com/indepth/2020/6/7/21258676/coronavirus-utah-nursing-homes-long-term-care-pandemic-covid-19-assisted-living-death-cna-nurses. Accessed 2020.
3. Assistant Secretary for Public Affairs (ASPA), CARES act provider relief fund: data. HHS.gov. Available at: https://www.hhs.gov/coronavirus/cares-act-provider-relief-fund/data/index.html. Accessed 2021.
4. Flinn B. States Leverage Medicaid to Provide Nursing Homes a Lifeline through COVID-19. Available at: https://leadingage.org/regulation/states-leverage-medicaid-provide-nursing-homes-lifeline-through-covid-19. Accessed 2021.
5. Harrington C, Schnelle JF, McGregor M, et al. Article commentary: the need for higher minimum staffing standards in U.S. nursing homes. Health Serv Insights 2016;9:13–9. https://doi.org/10.4137/hsi.s38994.
6. Gorges RJ, Konetzka RT. Staffing levels and COVID-19 cases and outbreaks in U.S. nursing homes. J Am Geriatr Soc 2020;68(11):2462–6. https://doi.org/10.1111/jgs.16787.
7. Appropriateness of minimum nurse staffing ratios in nursing homes. Report to congress: phase II final, vol 1. Prepared by Abt Associates Inc. Available at: https://theconsumervoice.org/uploads/files/issues/CMS-Staffing-Study-Phase-II.pdf. Accessed December 24, 2001.

8. Li Y, Temkin-Greener H, Shan G, et al. COVID-19 infections and deaths among connecticut nursing home residents: facility correlates. J Am Geriatr Soc 2020; 68(9):1899–906. https://doi.org/10.1111/jgs.16689.

9. Centers for Disease Control and Prevention. FastStats - nursing home care. Centers for Disease Control and Prevention. Available at: https://www.cdc.gov/nchs/fastats/nursing-home-care.htm. Accessed March 1, 2021.

10. Quality care for nursing home residents and workers during COVID–19 and beyond act, H.R. 598, 117th congress. 2021. Available at: https://www.congress.gov/bill/117th-congress/house-bill/598/text.

11. Quality care for nursing home residents act, S.315, 117th congress. Available at: https://www.congress.gov/bill/117th-congress/senate-bill/315/all-info. Accessed 2021.

12. Average registered nurse (RN) with long term care skills hourly pay. PayScale. Available at: https://www.payscale.com/research/US/Job=Registered_Nurse_(RN)/Hourly_Rate/f84e31c5/Long-Term-Care.

13. Average Registered Nurse (RN) With long term care skills hourly pay. Available at: https://www.payscale.com/research/US/Job=Registered_Nurse_(RN)/Hourly_Rate/f84e31c5/Long-Term-Care.

14. Certified Nurse's Assistant - Nursing Home Salary in the United States (n.d.). Long Term Care Facility Nursing Assistant Salaries in the United States. Indeed.com. Available at: https://www.indeed.com/cmp/Long-Term-Care-Facility/salaries/Nursing-Assistant.

15. NAB's brand is recognized as the authority for leadership core competencies in long term care. National Association of Long Term Care Administrator Boards. (n.d.). Available at: https://www.nabweb.org/about-us.

16. *How to become a licensed nursing home* administrator. MHA Online. Available at: https://www.mhaonline.com/faq/how-do-i-become-a-nursing-home-administrator.

17. Beth C, Mary E C, Shari T. Strengthening nurse leadership in long-term care: a case study. J Geriatr Med Gerontol 2018;4(3). https://doi.org/10.23937/2469-5858/1510051.

18. Blanchard K. Servant leadership: a new approach to creating a culture of success. The Ken Blanchard Companies; 2020. Available at: https://resources.kenblanchard.com/servant-leadership/servant-leadership-perspectives.

Dementia-Specific Nursing Care Competencies for Nursing Education and Long-Term Care Practice

Ann M. Mayo, RN, DNSc, FAAN

KEYWORDS

- Nursing competency • Neurodegenerative dementia disease • Care management
- Caregiver

KEY POINTS

- Dementia is a life-limiting condition requiring an extensive amount of complicated care.
- Dementia-specific nursing care can support both the person living with dementia as well as their caregivers.
- Eight dementia-specific care competencies are presented in this article.
- Nursing faculty and nurse leaders in long-term care have opportunities to incorporate dementia-specific nursing care competencies into the education of their students and their own and other nurses' practice.

OVERVIEW

Enhanced dementia-specific nursing care is needed for the rapidly expanding population of persons living with dementia (PLWD) across all settings, including long-term care (LTC) settings such as nursing homes. While a number of national nursing organizations have endorsed broader geriatric and aging nursing competencies, dementia-specific competencies have not received the same level of attention. The time is now to re-evaluate geriatric nursing competencies currently being used in academia as well as in practice settings. Dementia nursing care competencies should be incorporated into the current curricula for prelicensure RN programs and postlicensure RN programs (eg, MSN, postmasters, DNP) as well as in LTC job descriptions and annual competency programs. Like all competencies, these competencies serve as the basis for academic nursing faculty and practice settings leaders to develop specific measurable objectives that ensure effective, safe, and high-quality outcomes for PLWD. This article proposes a set of eight dementia-specific nursing care

Hahn School of Nursing & Health Science, Beyster Institute of Nursing Research, University of San Diego, 5998 Alcala' Park, San Diego, CA 92110, USA
E-mail address: Amayo@sandiego.edu

Nurs Clin N Am 57 (2022) 217–232
https://doi.org/10.1016/j.cnur.2022.02.004
nursing.theclinics.com

competencies. In addition, recognizing that some academic faculty and nurse leaders may be less familiar with dementia and dementia-specific care management, overviews are also provided on current scientific findings for Alzheimer's disease and the related dementias (ADRD), the Progressively Lowered Stress Theory (PLST), and person-centered care (PCC). Competency and care delivery examples will be provided in the context of the nursing home setting due to the concentrated population of PLWD in that setting.

BACKGROUND

Nursing is a practice discipline. To understand if nurses are delivering effective, high-quality, cost-effective care, nursing practice must be evaluated. Competencies serve as important guideposts for ensuring that safe and appropriate nursing care is being delivered to patients. Evaluating nurse competencies is important in academic and health care delivery settings, especially in nursing homes where 64.1 to 66.9% of residents have recently been reported to have dementia making them a vulnerable population.[1,2] Identifying and measuring nurses' abilities to plan, deliver and evaluate care constitute the function of professional competencies within the discipline. Using a competency framework allows specific domains to organize the competencies. For example, Hoke[3] identified three domains: Knowledge, Attitudes, and Skills. Knowledge represents the nurse's comprehension of what is important underpinning practice, attitudes represent knowing how to judge, choose, make a decision and act, and skills represent practice expertise.[4] These three competency domains provide a framework for specific objectives to be developed and measured appropriately.

Nurse competencies can also be differentiated based on a variety of criteria such as education level, type of license/certification, or specialty. For example, competency topics and levels of measurement may differ for students, registered nurses (RN), and advanced practice nurses (APNs). Competencies for RN directors of nursing in LTC might include the ability to design, maintain and assess a comprehensive communication plan for interactions between staff, residents, and family members. Competencies for APNs might include *advanced* assessments, diagnostic procedures, and treatments. Finally, competencies can be measured as met or not met; but can also be evaluated on a hierarchical scale such as *demonstrating the skill with at least 2 cues, demonstrating the skill only with only 1 cue,* or *consistently demonstrating the skill, no cueing.*

COMPETENCY-BASED AGING NURSING CARE

Caring for older adults has relevance for many practicing nurses.[5] Therefore, competencies that measure nurse knowledge, attitudes, and skills when nurses care for older adults is important. Excellent sources for aging competencies have been developed by a number of nursing organizations.[6] For example, a comprehensive listing of resources covering gerontological nursing competencies for different settings such as acute care hospitals and a range of roles such as RNs and APNs is included in the Gerontological Nursing: Scope and Standards of Practice.[7]

The collaborative work of many professional nursing specialty organizations such as the American Association of Nurse Practitioners and National Association of Clinical Nurse Specialists, funded by the Atlantic Philanthropies and overseen by the Nurse Competence in Aging (NCA) program, started in the 2000s. This coordinated effort began by targeting practicing nurses who were members of nursing specialty organizations, 20% of the practicing nurses in the US at the time. Next, the American Association of Colleges of Nursing (AACN) entry-to-practice aging competencies, some of which were developed as part of the NCA program, targeted academic degree programs. While it is outside the scope of this article to present all of these aging competencies, a few of those competencies relevant to the care of PLWD are provided in **Table 1**. In the table, the sample nurse aging competency statements are differentiated by BSN-prepared RN and two APN categories (Adult-Gerontology Clinical Nurse Specialist and Adult-Gerontology Nurse Practitioner) as reflected the AACN documents.[8–10]

DEMENTIA

Dementia is a public health crisis around the world affecting LTC as well as many other settings where older adults reside. There are approximately 50 million PLWD world-wide and costs of care for this life-limiting condition are well over $1 trillion dollars per year worldwide.[11] At the same time, much has been learned about the biology of ADRD over the past decade. For example, because a confirmatory diagnosis for AD can only be determined at autopsy, a biological definition using the presence or absence of amyloid and tau proteins measured via neuroimaging is now available.[12,13]

While advancements in dementia science are exciting, ADRD treatments remain elusive and dementia continues to be a life-limiting condition.[14] Therefore, PLWD experience an unrelenting downward trajectory in cognition (eg, memory, executive function, attention) that affects their ability to function independently. Not surprising, instrumental activities of daily living such as managing finances are compromised in the early stage culminating in severe impairments in basic activities of daily living such as bathing and feeding oneself.[14] Unfortunately, PLWD are at risk for many un-toward events such as falls, pneumonia, and delirium across all settings (eg, home, hospital, nursing homes).[15] Strong nursing leadership by competent RNs is needed in LTC to design systems of care that prevent such events.

CARING FOR PERSONS LIVING WITH DEMENTIA

Many of the PLWD reside in nursing homes. And while there are various staff members who have responsibilities for specific aspects of care, the accountability of caring for these PLWD falls squarely on the shoulders of the RN nurse leaders, many of whom are the nursing directors.

Several aspects need to be taken into consideration when designing and imple-menting quality care for PLWD. One aspect is that there are three different stages of ADRD disease (mild, moderate, and severe) (**Table 2**).[16] Not every nursing home resident with dementia will be admitted in the severe stage, many will develop demen-tia during their time as a resident. Discovering associations between these stages, be-haviors, and functional status has allowed for the design of stage-specific interventions for PLWD. Additionally, the FDA has determined that some pharmaceu-ticals such as cholinesterase inhibitors be prescribed based on the stage.[17] Therefore, dementia stage is an important consideration for designing care and treatments.

A second aspect to consider when caring for PLWD is that there are different related dementia subtypes. Presentations of each subtype can be very distinct, especially early on in the disease process. The most common neurodegenerative dementia sub-types include AD, frontotemporal dementia (FTD) and related syndromes, and Lewy body dementia (LBD). Each has a specific type of abnormal neurodegenerative pro-teinopathy that causes different symptoms over the course of the disease. Amyloid-B as in AD or alpha-synuclein as in LBD is examples of different proteins.[18] Symptoms, especially early on in the disease, include primarily memory problems for those with AD and personality changes for those with FTD. All PLWD will eventually display symptoms of distress such as wandering or refusing care.

Table 1		
Examples of AACN baccalaureate and advanced practice adult-gerontology competencies		
Type of Nursing Program	**Sample Competency Statement**	**Reference**
Baccalaureate	Implement and monitor strategies to prevent risk and promote quality and safety (eg, falls, medication mismanagement, pressure ulcers) in the nursing care of older adults with physical and cognitive needs.[a]	AACN, 2010, pg. 12
Adult-Gerontology Clinical Nurse Specialist	Develops evidence-based clinical interventions and systems to achieve defined patient and systems outcomes.[b]	AACN, 2010, pg. 14
Adult-Gerontology Acute Care Nurse Practitioner competency statement	Prescribes and monitors treatments and therapeutic devices as indicated, including but not limited to: oxygen, bi-level PAP, prosthetics, splints, and adaptive equipment.[c]	AACN, 2012, pg. 19

Abbreviations: AACN, American Association of Colleges of Nursing
   [a] AACN (2010)[8].
   [b] AACN (2010)[9].
   [c] AACN (2012)[10].

The cause of symptoms of distress is an additional aspect to consider in the care of PLWD. Symptoms of distress such as agitation among PLWD can interfere with the delivery of safe and effective nursing care.[19] These symptoms are associated with the expected progressive decline in cognitive abilities. These symptoms of distress result from an increasing perception by the PLWD that stressful stimuli are growing in intensity[20] and complexity and are now outside of their control. In other words, experiences that earlier in the disease process did not produce stress, now do. This lowered stress threshold causes the PLWD to be overly sensitive to situations resulting in problematic (for the staff) symptoms being more prevalent over time.[19] Staff can be taught to identify environmental triggers (eg, bathing too early in the day causes agitation) to make environmental modifications (eg, changing bath time) thereby decreasing the behavioral symptom of distress.[21–23]

A final consideration in the design of care for PLWD is person-centered care (PCC) planning. This approach to care can be implemented by nursing home staff to control situations that trigger the intensifying stress. PCC is an important approach to providing care for the PLWD. The American Geriatrics Society (AGS)[24] defines PCC as health care that is informed and guided by an individuals' expressed values and preferences. Collaboration with the individual, others important to the individual, and health care professionals informs the care decision-making to the extent that the individual wishes.[24] PCC interventions use a sociopsychological treatment approach focusing on the individuality of the person. Health care providers, after understanding more about the PLWD, can better target unmet needs in the context of the PLWD's history. For example, understanding that the PLWD previously bathed before dinner, planning care accordingly in a new long-term care setting could reduce agitation during bath time. PCC planning has also demonstrated decreased neuropsychiatric symptoms and depression, and improved well-being and quality of life.[25]

Table 2			
Type and level of compromise categorized by stage of dementia			
	Dementia Stage		
Type of Compromise	**Mild**	**Moderate**	**Severe**
Cognition	Slight (eg, memory lapses)	Modest (eg, missing appointments)	Confusion Lack of awareness of surroundings
Functional Status	IADLs: Slight ADLs: Intact	IADLs: Modest ADLs: Slight (eg, needs assistance with bathing)	Dependent on caregivers
Bowel and Bladder	Intact	Beginning to slight decline	Dependent on caregivers
Participation in Activities	Intact to slight decline	Slight to modest decline	Dependent on caregivers
Decisional Capacity	Intact	Slight to modest decline	Dependent on caregivers or legal guardians
Impact upon Caregiver	Worrisome	Increasing burden (eg, respite recommended)[a,b]	Increasing burden (eg, 24-h care required, hospice care recommended)[a,c]

Course of disease may be dependent upon dementia subtype.
[a] Alzheimer's Association.[51].
[b] Monson.[59].
[c] Regier, Hodgson, Gotlin[16].

Recognizing that dementia is a progressive life-limiting disease, the PLWD needs will change and may at times even be unpredictable. Therefore, PCC interventions need to be adapted as the disease progresses.[25]

COMPETENCY-BASED NURSING DEMENTIA CARE

Due to the high number of older PLWD, it is imperative that nurses in LTC, no matter their academic degree of preparation, can provide, coordinate and lead in the provision of high-quality dementia care to PLWD who are in different dementia stages and have different dementia subtypes. The amount of direct care versus coordination of care versus leadership may differ depending upon nurse preparation (degree and experience), role (RN vs APN), practice setting, staffing levels, actual staff availability, and of course the PLWD's assessment.

High-quality nursing dementia-specific care requires nurses to demonstrate knowledge, attitudes, and/or skills in the 8-core competencies presented in **Box 1**. Nurse faculty in schools of nursing and RNs and APNs in LTC would use each core competency to develop a separate set of measurable objectives. Measuring these objectives would determine if a student or nurse had met the core competency. Each objective could be differentiated for RNs versus APNs. For example, a specific objective for prescribing medications would be applicable for APNs but would not be listed as an objective for RNs. Or, objectives could be written for both roles and then the categories of measurement would be comprehensive enough to apply to both RNs and APNs. For example, regarding multidisciplinary planning meetings, the options could include "no involvement" to "arranges meeting" to "participates in meeting" to "leads meeting." Demonstrating competence for an RN may be "arranges meeting" while for an APN the expectation would be "leads meeting."

The first core competency, *Neurodegenerative Dementia Disease*, underpins all subsequent competencies. Without an understanding of the degenerative nature of neurological-based dementia and the dementia subtypes, limited individualized care planning can be provided to PLWD or their families. For example, would a greater focus be placed on assessing for risks due to memory loss or impaired decision-making if a PLWD had mild FTD versus AD? Because of the initial location of abnormal protein build-up in the brain, mild FTD results in earlier impaired decision-making compared to AD. Therefore, the person with FTD and family members should be made alert to possible financial issues related to poor decision-making such as giving money or other valuable possessions to staff. On the other hand, a PLWD who had a recent diagnosis of AD would have early memory problems, possibly not remembering a new staff person, and benefitting from repetitive introductions for the first week or so.

In all practice settings, including LTC settings such as nursing homes, nurses should be prepared to screen their patients for cognitive (memory and thinking) problems to determine if referrals for more comprehensive exams are needed.[26] Three available screening (not diagnostic) instruments that have demonstrated reliability and produce valid data are the Folstein Mini-Mental State Exam (MMSE),[27] Montreal Cognitive Assessment[28] and AD8.[29] Screening is important to determine if a resident needs follow-up to determine a diagnosis for optimal care planning. For example, a psychiatric mental health nurse practitioner may refer a resident with new memory problems to a neurology team for a more comprehensive exam that is targeted to diagnose a specific neurodegenerative disease.

In addition, nurses need an understanding that all neurodegenerative dementias are life-limiting serious illness conditions. It is important to note that palliative care is distinct from hospice care.[30] This understanding would better ensure palliative care services are offered at the time of a dementia diagnosis, not just when the PLWD needs hospice-level care. When doing so early, PLWD, family members, and staff will have the support to navigate through each stage of dementia, maintaining the highest quality of life possible for the PLWD.

Communication & Shared Decision-making, the second core competency, acknowledges the PLWD and family as important and integral in the planning of dementia care.[30] Communication between nurses, staff, PLWD, and family members is needed early on to ensure education and support are provided throughout the course of dementia. Without PLWD (when able) and family input, care is more difficult to individualize.[31] Multidisciplinary planning meetings are especially important in the nursing home setting.

Care and planning decisions can often be difficult for families without bidirectional communication and shared decision-making with health care professionals. For families living out of the area, technology can substantially improve communication[32] and shared decision-making between nurses and family members, especially when the PLWD is a resident in a nursing home. While there is acknowledgment of the difficulties of maintaining shared decision-making with the PLWD in the context of severe dementia, training of health care professionals in shared decision-making processes has demonstrated improved family decision-making with less family decisional conflict in the long term.[33] As patient and family advocates, nurses are perfectly positioned to lead multidisciplinary teams that emphasize communication and shared decision-making.

Box 1
Core competencies, sample objectives, and resources

Core Competency #1

Neurodegenerative Dementia Disease

Sample Objectives

"Demonstrates the ability to ..."
1. Identify dementia subtype and severity level (K)
2. Screen older adults for cognitive impairment (K, S)

Resources
- Husain, M. & Schott, J. M. (2016). Oxford University Press. Oxford Textbook of Cognitive Neurology and Dementia. SBN: 9,780,199,655,946
- Elahi, & Miller, B. (2017). A clinicopathological approach to the diagnosis of dementia. *Natures Review Neurology, 13*(8):457 to 476. doi: 10.1038/nrneurol.2017.96.
- Galvin, J. E. & Zweig, Y. (2018). The AD8: The Washington University Dementia Screening Test. https://hign.org/sites/default/files/2020-06/Try_This_Dementia_14.pdf
- Mezy, M. & Maslow, K. (2016). Recognition of dementia in hospitalized older adults. (Video also available on site). https://hign.org/consultgeri/try-this-series/recognition-dementia-hospitalized-older-adults

Core Competency #2
Communication & Shared Decision-making

Sample Objectives
"Demonstrates the ability to ..."
1) Involve PWD (mild Alzheimer's disease) and family members in the development of plan of care (K, A)
2) Lead multidisciplinary, (including family) planning meeting for nursing home placement of PWD (severe dementia) (K, A, S)

Resources
- Maslow, K. Mezey, M. & Hall, G. R. (2016). Working with families of hospitalized older adults with dementia. (Video also available on site). https://hign.org/consultgeri/try-this-series/working-families-hospitalized-older-adults-dementia
- Salmond, S. W. & Echevarria, M. (2017). Healthcare transformation and changing roles for nurses. *Orthopedic Nursing, 36*(1), 12 to 25.
- Hirschman, K. B. et al (2015). Continuity of care: The Transitional care model. The Online Journal of Issues in Nursing, 20(3). https://ojin.nursingworld.org/MainMenuCategories/ANAMarketplace/ANAPeriodicals/OJIN/TableofContents/Vol-20 to 2015/No3-Sept-2015/Continuity-of-Care-Transitional-Care-Model.html

Core Competency #3
Supportive Care Management for IADLs (mild to moderate dementia)

Sample Objectives
"Demonstrates the ability to ..."
1) Recommend to PWD and family financial support services based on dementia subtype and severity (K, S)
2) Provide resources to PWD and family to access state driving recommendations (K, S)

Resources
- NIH (2020). Financial problems can be the first sign of dementia onset. https://www.nih.gov/news-events/nih-research-matters/financial-problems-can-be-sign-dementia-onset
- Alzheimer's Association (2021). Financial and legal planning for caregivers. https://www.alz.org/help-support/caregiving/financial-legal-planning
- Fraade-Blanar, L. A. et al (2019). Diagnosed dementia and the risk of motor vehicle crash among older drivers. https://www.ncbi.nlm.nih.gov/pmc/articles/PMC5869102/pdf/nihms937962.pdf
- Accident Analysis & Prevention 113, 47 to 53. https://doi.org/10.1016/j.aap.2017.12.021

- Dementia Care Central (2019). Driving & dementia/State laws, coping and advice for caregivers. https://www.dementiacarecentral.com/caregiverinfo/driving-problems/

Core Competency #4
Supportive Care Management for Basic ADLs (severe dementia)

Sample Objectives
"Demonstrates the ability to ..."
1) Assess PWD swallowing using organizational nursing protocol (S)
2) Respect PWD privacy during the delivery of ADL support (A)

Resources
- Batchelor-Murphy, M. & Amella, E. J. (2019). Eating and feeding issue in older adults with dementia. Part I & II. (Videos also available on sites). Part I: https://hign.org/consultgeri/try-this-series/eating-and-feeding-issues-older-adults-dementia-part-i-assessment Part II: https://hign.org/consultgeri/try-this-series/eating-and-feeding-issues-older-adults-dementia-part-ii-interventions
- Scales, K., Zimmerman, S. & Miller, S. J. (2018). Evidence-Based Nonpharmacological Practices to Address Behavioral and Psychological Symptoms of Dementia. Gerontologist, 58(Suppl 1), S88–S102. https://www.ncbi.nlm.nih.gov/pmc/articles/PMC5881760/

Core Competency #5
Supportive Care Management for Symptoms of distress

Sample Objectives
"Demonstrates the ability to ..."
1) Identify most prevalent symptoms of distress attributed to Alzheimer's disease (K)
2) Ensure a safe environment for PWD who wander (K,S)

Resources
- Scales, K., Zimmerman, S. & Miller, S. J. (2018). Evidence-Based Nonpharmacological Practices to Address Behavioral and Psychological Symptoms of Dementia. Gerontologist, 58(Suppl 1), S88–S102. https://www.ncbi.nlm.nih.gov/pmc/articles/PMC5881760/
- Lach, H. W. (2019). Home safety inventory for older adults with dementia. *Try This:* Series: Best practice in nursing care to older adults. Hartford Institute for Geriatric Nursing, NYU Rory Meyers College of Nursing. Available at https://hign.org/consultgeri/try-this-series/home-safety-inventory-older-adults-dementia
- Silverstein, N. M. (2020). Wandering in the hospitalized older adult. (Video also available on site). *Try This:* Series: Best practice in nursing care to older adults. Hartford Institute for Geriatric Nursing, NYU Rory Meyers College of Nursing. Available at https://hign.org/consultgeri/try-this-series/wandering-hospitalized-older-adult

Core Competency #6
Risk Assessment for Adverse Outcomes

Sample Objectives
"Demonstrates the ability to ..."
1) Use the Confusion Assessment Method (CAM) to identify delirium (K, S)
2) Assess for Central Nervous System-active polypharmacy and report to prescriber (K)

Resources
- Sharon K. Inouye, S. K. Jones, R. N. & Marcantonio,E. R. (2020). Screening for delirium with the Confusion Assessment Method (CAM).
- https://deliriumnetwork.org/screening-for-delirium-with-the-confusion-assessment-method/
- Maust, D. T., Kim, H. M., Chiang, C. & Helen C. Kales, H. C. (2018). Association of the centers for Medicare & Medicaid Services national partnership to improve dementia care with the use of antipsychotics and other psychotropics in long-term care in the United States from 2009 to 2014. JAMA Internal Medicine, 178(5), 640–647. doi: 10.1001/jamainternmed.2018.0379

Core Competency #7
Palliative Care and Advance Directives

Sample Objectives

"Demonstrates the ability to …"
1) At time of dementia diagnosis refer PWD & families for palliative care services (K,A,S)
2) Inform PWD and family members of the health directive for dementia (University of Washington) (K,S)

Resources
- Harris D. (2007). Forget me not: palliative care for people with dementia. *Postgraduate Medical Journal, 83*(980), 362 to 366. https://doi.org/10.1136/pgmj.2006.052936
- Mitchell, S. L., Teno, J. M., Kiely, D. K., et al. (2009). The clinical course of advanced dementia. New England Journal of Medicine, *361*, 1529 to 1538.
- Gaster, Larson & Curtis (2017). Advance directives for dementia: Meeting a unique challenge. *JAMA,* 318(22), 2175 to 2176. https://doi.org/10.1001/jama.2017.16473
- University of Washington (n. d.). Advance directive for dementia. https://dementia-directive. org

Core Competency #8
Caring for the Caregiver

Sample Objectives
"Demonstrates the ability to …"
1) Assess for caregiver burden (K,S)
2) Refer caregivers to appropriate type of respite services (eg, in home, daycare center) (S)

Resources
- Peipert, J. D., Jennings, L. A., Hays, R. D., Wenger, N. S., Keeler, E. & Reuben, D. B. (2018). A Composite Measure of Caregiver Burden in Dementia: The Dementia Burden Scale-Caregiver. *Journal of the American Geriatrics Society, 66*(9), 1785 to 1789.
- Alzheimer's Association (2021). Respite care. https://www.alz.org/help-support/caregiving/care-options/respite-care
- NASEM (2021). Meeting the challenge of caring for persons with dementia and their care partners and caregivers: A way forward. (see Prologue for sample case study content)

Abbreviations: A, attitudes; K, knowledge; S, skills.

The third core competency is *Supportive Care Management for Instrumental Activities of Daily Living* (IADL) (mild to moderate dementia). An important component of this third core competency is the ability to recognize when and how IADLs can become compromised earlier on in dementia such as in mild and moderate stages. Residents may be in a nursing home long term for physical impairment and develop dementia after they became a resident. For example, the inability of a person with early FTD to make sound financial decisions would necessitate that someone, in addition to the PLWD, be present during financial transactions. Such decisions reinforce that the two previous competencies underpin this third competency.

The fourth core competency, *Supportive Care Management for Basic ADLs* addresses care for persons with severe dementia who are encountered most frequently in LTC settings, especially nursing homes. Examples of basic ADL include feeding, bathing, and mobility. Nursing skills for this competency may include the ability to assess a nursing home resident's swallowing. While nurses may not always be directly providing ADL to the PLWD, they are responsible for ensuring that care is individualized, safe, and being delivered in a respectful and caring manner. As an example, nursing home bathing should be in a private setting and if residents must be moved to the central location for bathing, they should be clothed appropriately during the transport. Routine ADL care should be individualized as much as possible[24] with nurses designing systems of care to assist staff in delivering high-quality care.

Supportive Care Management for Symptoms of Distress, the fifth core competency, nicely illustrates a synthesis of knowledge between dementia, PLST, and PCC.

Symptoms of distress typically arise because of a perceived stressor in the environment many times causing agitation in the PLWD.[34] Stress triggers may even include the style of approach of a nurse or staff person.[35] Symptoms of distress behaviors include aggressive psychomotor and nonpsychomotor behaviors, verbally aggressive behaviors and passive behaviors such as apathy[36] and can begin in any of the stages of dementia. Specific examples include wandering, yelling, and hitting. Nurses should begin with nonpharmacological approaches[37] such as distraction activities and therapeutic activity kits[38] that are of interest to the PLWD to prevent or break the cycle of behaviors.

Nurses should always conduct a thorough assessment of the PLWD and the environment to identify the cause of the behavior. For example, assessing for pain is important, especially in PLWD in nursing homes who are in the severe stage and unable to speak. The Hartford Institute for Geriatric Nursing *Try This: Series* of assessments and best practice approaches to care for older adults includes a pain assessment for PLWD.[39] Characteristics of the social and physical environment may also cause symptoms of distress.[37] For example, loud noises can be a stressful trigger so resident rooms may need to changed.[40,41] As an advocate for PLWD and families, nurses should lead efforts to manage stressful environments.

Risk Assessment for Adverse Outcomes is the sixth core competency topic. Adverse outcomes for PLWD include delirium, urinary tract infections, dehydration, electrolyte imbalances, pneumonia, falls (with and without fractures) and polypharmacy.[42–44] Transitions between facilities such as a nursing home and a hospital (and back) are especially risky for PLWD. Handoffs from LTC settings to hospitals need to be planned for and access to up-to-date documentation must be available to all involved.[45] Not surprisingly, hospital stays can be complicated and even be up to 10 days longer for PLWD compared to those who do not have dementia,[46,47] suggesting that in-patient hospitals may be the least prepared of all health care settings to manage the care needs of PLWD.

It is especially important for PLWD, families, and all health care organizations that nurses, no matter the setting, are prepared to conduct risk assessments, and where risk prevention evidence exists, the processes are put into place. Risk assessments can be especially challenging, especially when the PLWD has communication difficulties[30] as are encountered in the severe stage of dementia. An extensive array of older adult *Try This: Series* assessments and prevention plans (eg, delirium) targeting PLWD are available on the Hartford Institute for Geriatric Nursing website.[48] Recognizing that comprehensive care management is needed, the nursing role includes coordinating interprofessional collaborative teams so that comprehensive risk assessments are completed by responsible healthcare professionals.

The seventh core competency topic is *Palliative Care and Dementia-Specific Advance Directive*. Palliative care is a holistic approach to care provided to patients and families. While support too often begins only when a patient is at the end of life, palliative care ideally begins at the point in time it is determined that a patient has a life-limiting condition. This is emphasized here because AD and the related dementia subtypes are life-limiting conditions. Nurses should be prepared to make referrals to palliative care teams,[30] participate in team meetings, and in a more advanced specialty role, lead palliative care teams.

To proactively facilitate health care decision-making an advance directive is important. In the context of dementia care, nurses should be knowledgeable of the Dementia-Specific Advance Directive.[49] This directive is a supplement to any other health care advance directives PLWD may possess. Developed by a University of Washington multidisciplinary team, this dementia-specific advance directive is a multipage form that queries a person before they have dementia about four important goals of care (prolonging life, undergoing treatments to prolong life, being transferred to a higher level of care, and receiving only comfort care). Unique to this process, these four goals are queried about three times; each in the context of possibly having mild dementia, moderate dementia, and severe dementia in the future. Nurses who are in roles that include either having discussions with patients and families or encouraging such discussions can use this advance directive to promote end-of-life conversations in the context of the three stages of dementia.[50]

Care of the Caregiver is the final core competency presented. In the US over 15 million caregivers are providing complex care to PLWD, mostly on their own before their care recipient becomes a nursing home resident.[51,52] Many of these care recipients will have been hospitalized just before their admission to the nursing home and may return to their home after rehabilitation. Unfortunately, only three out of five caregivers report ever receiving any care instructions when a family member is discharged from a hospital.[52] Because not all PLWD will live their lives out in a nursing home, nurses working in nursing homes should be prepared to counsel and educate caregivers to keep the PLWD out of institutions in the future.[53]

In addition, nurses need to be able to assess and monitor the caregiver's emotional and physical functional status; in other words, the possible burdensome toll of caregiving. Numerous caregiver burden instruments, such as the Caregiver Burden Inventory, measure physical, social and emotion effects of caregiving.[54,55] Once assessed, support services using agencies such as the Alzheimer's Association need to be coordinated. Respite services (that may involve bringing other family members), in-home professional care, daycare, and adaptations to the home environment may be needed to facilitate the work of the caregiver.

Research has demonstrated that not all aspects of caregiving experiences are negative; caregivers of PLWD have reported positive aspects as well. Examples include self-affirmation, high resilience, and a positive outlook on life; each known to be increased with higher perceived social, emotional, and informational support, and spirituality.[56–58] Identifying positive aspects of caregiving should be included in all caregiver assessments and then reaffirmed and reinforced with caregivers by nurses.[59]

RECOMMENDATIONS

While an ample supply of research-based literature supports the content of the eight competencies, future work is recommended. First, little is known about culturally informed dementia care. Issues likely exist as one study demonstrated that Hispanic PLWD were less likely to complete an advance directive.[60] More research investigating culturally focused dementia nursing care competencies is needed. This research trajectory would align with the National Institute of Nursing Research as articulated in the 2022 to 2026 draft Strategic Plan's first and second goals addressing "dismantling structures that perpetuate health disparities and impede health equity" and "social determinants of health across the lifespan" (NINR, p. 2).[61] Second, formally validating the competencies in samples of nursing students and practicing nurses, including APNs and across settings, including primary care, is also needed. Qualitative interviews using cognitive interviewing with nurses could be used to examine each of the competency topics as well as different measurement scales and response options.[62] Traditional tests of reliability and validity should also be conducted. Most importantly it should be determined if and how competencies are related to patient outcomes. For example, if nurses are competent in *care of the caregiver*, is the institutionalization of the PLWD avoided or at least delayed?

Maintaining faculty knowledge and skills in the care of older adults is the first competency included in the Competencies for Gerontological Nurse Educators.[63] That, coupled with the fact that gerontological nursing education currently covers a very wide range of topics, additional faculty expertise in some of the dementia-specific core competency topics may be needed to operationalize the dementia-specific competencies. Annual nursing and multi-disciplinary conferences such as presented by the Gerontological Advanced Practice Nurses Association and Gerontological Society of America offer sessions on dementia research and care topics. Organizations such as the Center to Advance Palliative Care offer on-line and in-person education specifically on care of PLWD.

Finally, nurse leaders in education and practice settings should advocate for and promote the use of dementia-specific nurse competencies to improve the quality of care for PLWD. The dementia-specific nurse competencies presented here are written so that they can be used to develop course objectives across all nursing programs (eg, entry level RN, APN). Deans of schools of nursing should support program directors in operationalizing the competencies that would include the use of a variety of settings such as nursing homes where students would have more frequent contact with PLWD. Directors of Nursing (DON) in nursing homes, who are responsible for the quality of resident care, employee job satisfaction and retention,[64] are likely aware of the importance of these competencies. However, they themselves may be burdened with administrative duties and have little time to maintain their own competency in nursing dementia care much less ensure staff maintain relevant competencies. Including the competencies in job descriptions and annual competency measurements will provide objective data to document the current level of competence required to make the case for increased staffing and training, if needed. Recognizing that the current Medicare nursing home payment system is flawed,[65] health care policy advocacy by nurses is needed to improve staffing, training of staff, and the numerous other financial issues encountered in nursing homes where many vulnerable PLWD reside.

SUMMARY

With over 50 million PLWD worldwide, dementia-specific nursing care has become critical for reducing the risks of adverse outcomes such as delirium and falls that are so common among this vulnerable population. Up to 66% of nursing home residents are estimated to have dementia.[66] Nurse competency required to safely care for these residents should include knowledge of dementia, skilled communication, shared decision-making, supportive care management for daily living experiences and symptoms of distress, and risk assessments. An important aspect of care delivery that is often overlooked is that palliative care services be instituted early in the disease, before end-of-life, because ADRD is life-limiting conditions. The proposed dementia-specific nursing care competencies, underpinned by PLST and PCC, aim to improve the quality of nursing care delivered to PLWD. Working together with PLWD, families, and multidisciplinary teams, nurses employed in LTC settings have the opportunity to improve the care experience and take the lead as experts in dementia care.

CLINICS CARE POINTS

- Operationalizing a PCC plan based on the resident's personal history can decrease symptoms of distress such as wandering and refusing care.
- As cognitive abilities decline overtime the resident's threshold for managing stress declines.

- Monitoring a resident's unique stress triggers and then adapting to the environment or situation can further reduce symptoms of distress.

DISCLOSURE

Author has no commercial or financial conflicts of interest. There are no funding sources for this work.

REFERENCES

1. Boscart VM, Sidani S, Poss J, et al. The associations between staffing hours and quality of care indicators in long-term care. BMC Health Serv Res 2018;18(1):750.
2. Cameron EJ, Bowles SK, Marshall EG, et al. Falls and long-term care: a report from the care by design observational cohort study. BMC Fam Pract 2018; 19(1):73.
3. Hoke MM, Robins LK. Continuing the cultural competency journey through exploration of knowledge, attitudes, and skills with advanced practice psychiatric nursing students: an exemplar. Nurs Clin North Am 2011;46:201–5.
4. Perez CFdA, Tourinho FSV, Junior PMC. Competencies in the nurse education process to care of the aging: an integrative review. Texto Contexto Enferm 2016;25(4):1–8. Accessed February 18, 2021.
5. Scholder J, Kagan S, Schumann MJ. Nurse competence in aging overview. Nurs Clin North Am 2004;39:429–42.
6. American Association of Colleges Nursing. American Association of Colleges of Nursing Curriculum Guidelines. 2021. Available at: https://www.aacnnursing.org/Education-Resources/Curriculum-Guidelines. Accessed March 3, 2021.
7. American Nurses Association. Gerontological nursing: scope and Standards. 2nd edition. Silver Spring: ANA, MD; 2019.
8. American Association of Colleges Nursing. Recommended Baccalaureate competencies and curricular guidelines for the nursing care of older adults: a supplement to the essentials of baccalaureate education for professional nursing practice. Washington (DC): AACN; 2010.
9. American Association of Colleges Nursing. Adult-gerontology clinical nurse specialist competencies. Washington (DC): AACN; 2010.
10. American Association of Colleges Nursing. Adult-gerontology acute care nurse practitioner competencies. Washington (DC): AACN; 2012.
11. Patterson C. World Alzheimer report state of the art of dementia research: new Frontiers. Alzheimer's Disease International; 2018. Available at: https://www.alzint.org/u/WorldAlzheimerReport2018.pdf. Accessed March 14, 2021.
12. Jack CR, Bennett DA, Blennow K, et al. NIA-AA research framework: toward a biological definition of Alzheimer's disease. Alzheimers Dement 2018;14(4): 535–62.
13. Therriault J, Benedet AL, Pascoal TA, et al. Frequency of biologically defined Alzheimer Disease in relation to age, sex, APOE e4, and cognitive impairment. Neurology 2021;96:e975–85.
14. Alzheimer's Association. Alzheimer's Association report: 2017 Alzheimer's disease facts and figures. Alzheimer's Demen 2017;13:325–73.
15. Young Y, Papenkov M, Hsu W, et al. Permanent transition of homecare recipients with dementia to nursing homes in New York state: Risk factors. Geriatr Nurs 2020;41:1–6.

16. Regier NG, Hodgson NA, Gitlin LN. Characteristics of activities for persons with dementia at the mild, moderate, and severe stages. Gerontologist 2017;57(5): 987–97.

17. Adlimoghaddam A, Neuendorff M, Roy B, et al. A review of clinical treatment considerations of donepezil in severe Alzheimer's disease. CNS Neurosci Ther 2018; 24(10):876–88.

18. Elahi FM, Miller B. A clinicopathological approach to the diagnosis of dementia. Nat Rev Neurol 2017;13(8):457–76.

19. Smith M, Gerdner LA, Hall GR, et al. History, development, and future of the progressively lowered stress threshold: a conceptual model for dementia care. J Am Geriatr Soc 2004;52:1755–60.

20. Stolley JM, Hall GR, Collins J, et al. Managing the care of patients with irreversible dementia during hospitalization for comorbidities. Nurs Clin North Am 1993;28(4): 767–82.

21. Chrabaszcz M. Preventing dysfunctional behaviors of those with dementia based on the progressively lowered threshold model. University of Massachusetts Amherst ScholarWorks@UMass Amherst. 2014. Available at: https://scholarworks. umass.edu/nursing_dnp_capstone. Accessed March 7, 2021.

22. Huang HL, Shyu YI, Chen MC, et al. A pilot study on a home-based caregiver training program for improving caregiver self-efficacy and decreasing the behavioral problems of elders with dementia in Taiwan. Int J Geriatr Psychiatry 2003;18: 337–45.

23. Robinson KM, Crawford TN, Buckwalter KC, et al. Outcomes of a two-component intervention on behavioral symptoms in persons with dementia and symptom response in their caregivers. J Appl Gerontol 2018;37(5):570–94.

24. American Geriatrics Society. Person-centered care: a definition and essential elements. The American Geriatrics Society Expert Panel on Person-Centered Care. 2015. Available at: https://doi-org.sandiego.idm.oclc.org/10.1111/jgs.13866 . Accessed March 10, 2021.

25. Kim SK, Park M. Effectiveness of person-centered care on people with dementia: a systematic review and meta-analysis. Clin Interv Aging 2017;12:381–97.

26. Maslow K, Fortinsky RH. Nonphysician care providers can help to increase detection of cognitive impairment and encourage diagnostic evaluation for dementia in community and residential care settings. Gerontologist 2018;58(S1): S20–31.

27. Folstein MF, Folstein SE, McHugh PR. Mini-mental state: a practical method for grading the cognitive state of patients for the clinician. J Psychiatr Res 1975; 12(3):189–98.

28. Finney GR, Minagar A, Heilman KM. Assessment of mental status. Neurol Clin 2016;34(1):1–16.

29. Galvin JE, Roe CM, Powlishta KK, et al. The AD8: a brief informant interview to detect dementia. Neurology 2005;65(4):559–64.

30. Molony SL, Kolanowski A, Van Haitsma K, et al. Person-centered assessment and care planning. Gerontologist 2018;58(S1):S32–47.

31. Maslow K, Mezey M, Hall GR. Working with families of hospitalized older adults with dementia. 2016. Available at: https://hign.org/consultgeri/try-this-series/ working-families-hospitalized-older-adults-dementia. Accessed March 4, 2021.

32. Witlatch CJ, Orsulic-Jeras S. Meeting the informational, educational, and psychosocial support needs of persons living with dementia and their family caregivers. Gerontologist 2018;58(S1):S58–73. Accessed March 4, 2021.

33. Giguere AMC, Lawani MA, Fortier-Brochu E, et al. Tailoring and evaluating an intervention to improve shared decision-making among seniors with dementia, their caregivers, and healthcare providers: study protocol for a randomized controlled trial. Trials 2018;19(332). Accessed March 4, 2021.

34. Halpern R, Seare J, Tong J, et al. Using electronic health records to estimate the prevalence of agitation in Alzheimer disease/dementia. Int J Geriatr Psychiatry 2019;34:420–31.

35. Galik E. When non-pharmacological approaches are not enough: Psychotropic medication management of neuropsychiatric symptoms of dementia. Gerontological Advanced Practice Nurses Association Virtual Annual Conference. 2020. Available at: https://library.gapna.org/gapna/sessions/1846/view. Accessed November 20, 2020.

36. Colling KB. A taxonomy of passive behaviors in people with Alzheimer's Disease. J Nurs Scholarsh 2020;32(3):239–44.

37. Scales K, Zimmerman S, Miller SJ. Evidence-Based Nonpharmacological practices to address behavioral and psychological symptoms of dementia. Gerontologist 2018;58(S1):S88–102.

38. McCabe D. Therapeutic activity kits. 2020. Available at: https://hign.org/consultgeri/try-this-series/therapeutic-activity-kits. Accessed March 4, 2021.

39. Horgas AL. Assessing pain in older adults with dementia. 2018. Available at: https://hign.org/consultgeri/try-this-series/assessing-pain-older-adults-dementia. Accessed March 4, 2021.

40. ACEP (n d. American College of Emergency Physicians Geriatric Emergency Accreditation. Available at: https://www.acep.org/globalassets/sites/geda/documnets/geda-criteria.pdf. Accessed March 2, 2021.

41. McClelland M, Sorrell JM. Enhancing Care of Older Adults in the Emergency Department. J Psychosoc Nurs Ment Health Serv 2015;53(3):18–21.

42. Harvey L, Mitchell R, Brodaty H, et al. The influence of dementia on injury-related hospitalisations and outcomes in older adults. Injury 2016;47(1):226–34.

43. Kao C, Lin C, Wu S, et al. Effectiveness of different memory training programs on improving hyperphagic behaviors of residents with dementia: a longitudinal single-blind study. Clin Intervaging 2016;11:707–20.

44. Reynish EL, Hapca SM, De Souza N, et al. Epidemiology and outcomes of people with dementia, delirium, and unspecified cognitive impairment in the general hospital: prospective cohort study of 10,014 admissions. BMC Med 2017;15(1):140.

45. Hirschman KB, Hodgson NA. Evidence-based interventions for transitions in care for individuals living with dementia. Gerontologist 2018;58(S1):S129–40.

46. Bernardes C, Massano J, Freitas A. Hospital admissions 2000–2014: A retrospective analysis of 288 096 events in patients with dementia. Arch Gerontol Geriatr 2018;77:150–7.

47. Motzek T, Werblow A, Tesch F, et al. Determinants of hospitalization and length of stay among people with dementia – An analysis of statutory health insurance claims data. Arch Gerontol Geriatr 2018;76:227–33.

48. John A. Hartford Institute for geriatric nursing. Hartford Institute for Geriatric Nursing; 2020. Available at: https://hign.org. Accessed March 4, 2021.

49. University of Washington (n.d. Advance Directive for Dementia. Available at: https://gim.uw.edu/news/barak-gaster-develops-dementia-specific-advance-directive. Accessed February 28, 2021.

50. Gaster B, Larson EB, Curtis JR. Advance directives for dementia: Meeting a unique challenge. JAMA 2017;318(22):2175–6.

51. Alzheimer's Association. Caregiving. Washington, DC: Alzheimer's Association. 2021. Available at: https://www.alz.org/help-support/caregiving?gclid=CjwKCAjw47eFBhA9EiwAy8kzNLbAP13ua4O0IAl8RLb1TT_EYrdG8osjNV1JD2JQsJdZ3m_FaYyP3xoC9r0QAvD_BwE. Accessed May 26, 2021.

52. Reinhard SC, Young HM, Levine C, et al. Home alone Revisited: family caregivers providing complex care. Washington (DC): AARP Public Policy Institute; 2019. Available at: https://www.aarp.org/content/dam/aarp/ppi/2019/04/home-alone-revisited-family-caregivers-providing-complex-care.pdf. Accessed July 3, 2019.

53. NASEM. Meeting the challenge of caring for persons with dementia and their care partners and caregivers: a way forward 2021. Available at: https://www.nap.edu/download/26026. Accessed May 1, 2021.

54. Novak M, Guest C. Application of a multidimensional caregiver burden inventory. Gerontologist 1989;29(6):798–803.

55. Valer DB, Aires M, Fengler FL, et al. Adaptation and validation of the caregiver burden inventory for use with caregivers of elderly individuals. Rev Lat Am Enfermagem 2015;23(1):130–8.

56. Hodge DR, Sun F. Positive feelings of caregiving among Latino Alzheimer's family caregivers: understanding the role of spirituality. Aging Ment Health 2012;16(6):689–98.

57. Jones SM, Edwards M, Mioshi E. Social support and high resilient coping in carers of people with dementia. Geriatr Nurs 2019;40(6):584–9.

58. Mayo AM, Siegle K, Savell E, et al. Lay caregivers' experiences with caring for persons with dementia: A phenomenological study. J Gerontol Nurs 2020;46(8):17–27.

59. Monson DA. Life satisfaction: aging Female informal caregivers of persons with dementia. San Diego (CA): University of San Diego; 2021. Available at: https://digital.sandiego.edu/dissertations/199/. Accessed on July 25, 2021.

60. Kwak J, Xie B, Champion JD, et al. Rural dementia caregivers in Southwest Texas: An exploratory study of advance directives and end-of-life proxy decision making. J Gerontol Nurs 2019;45(9):11–7.

61. National Institute of Nursing Research. National Institute of Nursing Research Strategic Plan Working Group Draft Framework for 2022-2026. Available at: https://www.ninr.nih.gov/sites/files/docs/strategic_planning_working_group_framework_report_051021_v1_508c.pdf. Accessed July 29, 2021.

62. Waltz CC, Strickland OL, Lenz ER. Measurement in nursing and health research. New York: Springer Publishing Company; 2017.

63. Wyman JF, Abdullah L, Baker N, et al. Development of core competencies and a recognition program for gerontological nurse educators. J Prof Nurs 2019;35(6):452–60.

64. Siegel EO, Young HM. Assuring quality in nursing homes: the black of administrative and clinical leadership-a scoping review. Gerontologist 2021;61(4):e147–62. Accessed July 25, 2021.

65. Harrington C, Dellefield ME, Halifax E, et al. Appropriate Nurse Staffing Levels for U.S. Nursing Homes. Health Serv Insights 2020;13. 1178632920934785.

66. Gaugler JE, Yu F, Davila HW, et al. Alzheimer's disease and nursing homes. Health Aff (Millwood) 2014;33(4):650–7.

Geropsychiatric Nursing Leadership in Long-Term Care

Pamela Z. Cacchione, PhD, CRNP, BC, FGSA, FAAN[a],*,
Wanda Spurlock, DNS, RN, GERO-BC, PMH-BC, CNE, FNGNA, ANEF[b],
Kathy Richards, PhD, RN, FAAN, FAASM[c], Melodee Harris, PhD, RN, FAAN[d]

KEYWORDS

- Nursing homes • Geropsychiatric nursing • Leadership • Dementia

KEY POINTS

- Geropsychiatric nursing (GPN) is a subspecialty.
- GPN leaders are essential to high-quality nursing home care.
- Initiatives to infuse GPN into undergraduate and graduate curricula, research and policy will prepare the next generation of GPN leaders.
- GPN leaders improve the care of older adults.

INTRODUCTION AND DEFINITION

Geropsychiatric nursing (GPN) has been defined by the GPN Collaborative[1,2] as the *holistic support for the care of older adults and their families as they anticipate and/ or experience developmental and cognitive challenges, mental health concerns, and psychiatric/substance misuse disorders across a variety of health and mental health care settings.*[1] The GPN Collaborative was started by a group of leaders in GPN, Drs Cornelia Beck, Kitty Buckwalter and Lois Evans funded by the John A Hartford Foundation to enhance the cognitive and mental health of older adults through Geropsychiatric Nurses.[3] This definition of GPN is purposively broad to encompass the integration of geropsychiatric care across the continuum of care.

The integration of GPN leadership into education, practice, research, and policy is essential to improve the quality of life of older adults living in long-term care settings. This has become gravely evident during the coronavirus disease-2019 (COVID-19) pandemic whereby older adults in long-term care were not only at

[a] University of Pennsylvania School of Nursing, 418 Curie Boulevard, Philadelphia, PA 19104, USA; [b] College of Nursing and Allied Health, Southern University and A&M College, J.K. Haynes Building, P.O. Box 11794, Baton Rouge, LA 70813, USA; [c] School of Nursing, University of Texas at Austin, 1710 Red River Street, Austin, TX 78712, USA; [d] College of Nursing, University of Arkansas for Medical Sciences, 4301 West Markham Street Slot #529, Little Rock, AR 72205, USA
* Corresponding author.
E-mail address: pamelaca@upenn.edu

Nurs Clin N Am 57 (2022) 233–244
https://doi.org/10.1016/j.cnur.2022.02.005
0029-6465/22/© 2022 Elsevier Inc. All rights reserved.
nursing.theclinics.com

risk physically from the virus but also at risk for several geropsychiatric conditions including depression, isolation, loneliness, exacerbation of the behavioral symptoms of dementia, psychosis, and suicide.[4] Geropsychiatric leadership in long-term care requires expert communication, motivation, and persuasion skills to improve the therapeutic environment and the uptake of evidence-based interventions for geropsychiatric conditions. Expert geropsychiatric assessments lead to evidence-based interventions that can improve the care and quality of life of older adults in long-term care. GPN leaders impact policy decisions and drive the long-term care research agenda.

History of Geropsychiatric Nursing Leadership

GPN leadership is needed in all settings but never more important than in the long-term care arena. Unfortunately, the workforce in long-term care is unprepared to meet the growing population of older adults with mental health conditions, especially in the nursing home.[5] To understand leadership in GPN in the nursing home, it is important to start at the beginning.

Dr Mary Starke Harper was the first geropsychiatric nurse and is considered the pioneer of GPN. Through her national and international leadership, she overcame many personal and professional obstacles to improve the quality of care for older adults with mental health disparities.[6] Dr Harper was born in 1919 in Alabama and was the first black woman to graduate from the University of Minnesota. She published many books and articles, became the first woman, black social scientist, established the Mary Starke Harper Geriatric Psychiatry Center, and mentored countless students. She was the first to call attention to mental health disparities for minority older adults and directed the National Institute of Mental Health Minority Fellowship program. Four United States Presidents looked to Dr Harper for advice on mental health and aging. She served on the Advisory Board for the National Institute of Aging and continued to work every day of her life until her death at 87 years old.[6]

GPN evolved rapidly under the leadership of Dr Mary Starke Harper. In the 1970s, GPN was a blended subspecialty shared between gerontological and psychiatric nurses. Clinical nurse specialists in gerontological or psychiatric mental health nursing took the first step toward blending the specialties in GPN.[7] During this same time frame, nurses certified in gerontological nursing also paved the way for future generations of geropsychiatric nurses by convening the first State of the Future Geropsychiatric Nursing Conference in 2005 took place in Philadelphia.[8] The National Invitational Geropsychiatric Nursing State of the Future Conference resulted in a series of white papers were published on GPN in the *Journal of the American Psychiatric Nursing* Association,[9] including a state of the science paper on GPN.[10]

Before her death in 2006, Dr Harper collaborated with geropsychiatric nurse leaders Jacqueline Stolley and Kathleen Buckwalter (1994) to publish results of a survey of geropsychiatric nurses.[11] The survey reported that geropsychiatric nurses held certifications in gerontological or psychiatric mental health nursing or both. The survey emphasized unity in the diversity within GPN. This survey identified problems that continue today such as lack of integrated or stand-alone curriculum in GPN, limited programs with courses in GPN focus. The survey showed that geropsychiatric nurses demonstrate "a diverse blend of skills" and recognized interprofessional roles of the geropsychiatric nurse. The survey respondents reported that their most important concern was the "recognition of the population.... that we serve." Geropsychiatric nurses strongly identified with persons living with dementia as the primary population with whom they worked, and they were very concerned about the quality of care in long-term care settings. The 1994 survey reported that GPN leaders prioritized recruitment and hiring of adequate nursing staff in long-term care, education of physicians, certification of staff, and the education and leadership training of staff.

Ten years later, in 2004, another survey by Kurlowicz and colleagues[12] (2007) concluded that there were few GPN programs and little integration of GPN content across graduate nursing specialties. In 2015, investigators conducted a follow-up national survey[13,14] and compared the results to earlier findings. They found little change in GPN content in graduate nursing education. Although there were more psychiatric nursing programs, GPN content continued to be embedded in the primary care curriculum, rather than psychiatric mental health curriculum.

In 2008, the Geropsychiatric Nursing Collaborative (GPNC) was led by Drs Cornelia Beck, Kathleen Buckwalter, and Lois Evans. The GPNC was housed in the American Academy of Nursing and funded by the John A Hartford Foundation. The purpose of the GPNC was to improve the cognitive and mental health of older adults by developing Geropsychiatric Nursing Competency Enhancements across all levels of nursing and to adapt, develop, and disseminate GPN curricula.[3,15]

In 2015, another Geropsychiatric Nursing State of the Future Conference was held in San Francisco. This conference used an interprofessional approach.[16] A series of white papers were published in a special issue of the Journal of the American Geriatrics Society.[17] The participants identified the need for a cadre of GPN leaders to define GPN, create curriculum, and enhance and grow the pipeline of geropsychiatric nurses, advanced practice nurses, and scientists. These geropsychiatric nurse leaders are positioned to: (1) engage professional organizations in addressing the lack of a certification examination for GPN, (2) form a leadership group for knowledge development, translation, and dissemination to improve quality of life for all older adults.[10]

In 2020, GPN leaders again supported the 1994 call for a wide range of specialties to include GPN within their scope of practice but most importantly for those who routinely care for older adults. The Gerontological Advanced Practice Nurses Association (GAPNA) Position Paper Supporting Evidence for Geropsychiatric Nursing as a Subspecialty of Gerontological Advanced Practice Nursing[19] supports within the discipline and interdisciplinary engagement in geropsychiatric care. Similar to the early survey of geropsychiatric nurses, the authors state the work of the diverse group of advanced practice nurses echoes the same passion to reflect "the highest respect and sensitivity for older adults and their families." The authors also used an interprofessional approach and continued a remarkable similarity in the recommendations of their predecessors to prioritize education and certification while making additional recommendations to improve the quality of life for diverse older adult populations.

Scope of Geropsychiatric Nursing Practice

GPN is a blend of many overlapping nursing roles.[20,21] Because, it is impossible to separate the mind from the body, at some point, it is likely that most nurses caring for older adults serve as geropsychiatric nurses, and those working in nursing homes do so daily. The overlapping of disciplines is very evident in the field of dementia care. For example, the Diagnostic and Statistical Manual of Mental Disorders[21] identify dementia as a psychiatric diagnosis. Yet according to the Centers for Disease Control and Prevention (CDC),[22] dementia is a term to describe memory loss. Alzheimer's disease-related dementia and vascular dementia are characterized as medical illnesses with discrete pathologic findings. In addition to depression and anxiety, a person living with dementia may also have a comorbid diagnosis of a severe and persistent mental illness such as schizophrenia or bipolar disorder.

Therefore, nurses who specialize in multiple disciplines, such as neurology, psychiatry, gerontology, and family practice, contribute to the care of persons living with dementia. Psychiatric mental health, family practice, adult-gerontology primary care, adult-gerontology acute care, and other gerontological advanced practice nurses may all practice, conduct research, and lead in long-term care settings. It is, therefore, critical that all nurses in long-term care receive training in GPN.[4]

Geropsychiatric Nursing Education

Despite the extraordinary efforts to improve the GPN curriculum, little is known about individual nurse practitioners', registered nurses', and licensed practical nurses' expertise and preparation to practice GPN in nursing homes. Although, more than 60% of the almost 1.5 million nursing employee FTEs are dedicated to employment in nursing homes,[23] only 11.9% of these employee FTEs are registered nurses.[23] This is a small number considering that the registered nurses are dispersed to more than 15,600 nursing homes and 1.3 million nursing home residents.[23] The COVID-19 pandemic highlighted the need for the 24-h presence of registered nurses in nursing homes to meet the psychosocial and physical needs of the older adults.[24]

Although there is no certification for GPN or long-term care for advanced practice registered nurses or registered nurses, GPN is a necessary subspecialty at the top of the Advanced Practice Registered Nursing Consensus Model[19] and best represents nursing leadership in the nursing home. Because of the nature of caring for older adults, the interprofessional team approach is not new to nursing homes and remains a foundational model of care for older adults.[24] Geropsychiatric nurses are well-positioned to lead interprofessional teams in US nursing homes.

GAPNA supports the subspecialty of GPN. Recommendations from the GAPNA position paper[19] for strengthening the subspecialty and GPN leaders include developing nursing competencies, integrating interprofessional education, removing scope of practice barriers, and endorsing a variety of strategies such as portfolio and educational development to support credibility for the scope of practice for this subspecialty.

Geropsychiatric Nursing Leadership

Meeting the health care needs of older adults in Nursing homes who live with dementia, psychiatric and substance use conditions poses challenges for GPN leadership. Recent data show that almost half (45%) of nursing home residents have a dementia diagnosis, while almost one-third (32%) have other psychiatric disorders such as schizophrenia, mood disorders, or other psychiatric diagnoses.[25] Of those with dementia, 61.4% had moderate to severe cognitive impairment.[26] Prevalence rates for Depression (46.3%) and delirium (15%–70%) provide further evidence for the pressing need for GPN expertise.[22,27] GPN leaders have the expertise to distinguish between these conditions, and this is exceedingly important because treatment plans for these conditions differ. Access to services and support for mental health needs, however, is often inadequate, especially for minority older adults in nursing homes who represent a growing proportion of that population.[28–30]

GPN leadership is particularly necessary when caring for older adults with dementia. Person-centered, evidence-based, nonpharmacological interventions are the frontline approaches for the treatment of behavioral and psychological symptoms of dementia. If nursing home clinicians are untrained, inconsistent, and unprepared to provide nonpharmacological interventions, antipsychotics may be prescribed. Therefore, the high turnover of certified nursing assistants and inadequate RN staffing pose significant barriers to reducing inappropriate use of antipsychotic medications putting residents at risk for adverse health outcomes.

Geropsychiatric nurse leaders must continue to engage in concerted efforts to influence evidence-based nursing practices and policy to improve the quality of care in nursing homes. The recognition and support of GPN as a subspecialty of gerontological advanced practice nursing is critical to filling the gap in the provision of comprehensive on-site geropsychiatric services and consultation in nursing homes, especially in rural and medically underserved areas whereby the demand for mental health providers exceeds the supply.[30] Moreover, advanced practice nurses specifically educated in GPN could play a key role in reducing the risk of potentially avoidable psychiatric hospitalizations, while supporting person-centered care planning and education and training of staff in dementia-related behavioral management approaches. An example of evidence-based strategies to support GPN leaders is the Nursing Home Toolkit (www.nursinghometoolkit.com/).[31] This web-based toolkit was funded by The Commonwealth Fund and The John A Hartford Foundation and provides evidence-based strategies to provide person-centered care for individuals exhibiting behaviors of psychological distress.

Although federal legislation has been proposed to amend titles XVIII (Medicare) and XIX (Medicaid) direct care to residents, including assessments, facilities are still only required to have one RN on site for 8 hours a day, regardless of the acuity and complexity of nursing home residents.[32,33] A group of 22 nursing gerontology and GPN experts recently called up the CMS Coronavirus Commission for Safety and Quality in Nursing Homes to enact policies to ensure appropriate 24-h RN coverage to guide the care provided to all older adults who reside in nursing homes.[24] "CMS oversight and more regulations cannot replace on the ground expert care and supervision provided by RNs."[24,26]

Exemplar of Geropsychiatric Nursing Leadership

Robust engagement of GPN leaders at local, state, and national levels is critical to improving LTC care. An example of proactive GPN leadership is the work of Dr Wanda Spurlock.

Dr Spurlock, through her past participation and leadership in the Louisiana Enhancing Aging with Dignity through Empowerment and Respect (LEADER), played a key role in Louisiana's reduction in antipsychotic medications in nursing homes. Dr Spurlock also served on the Louisiana Dementia Partnership, chaired the Advancing Excellence in America's Nursing Homes Special Interest Group, and was the contact to the CMS National Dementia Partnership.

In 2012, CMS established the *National Partnership to Improve Dementia Care in Nursing Homes*[33] in response to a report issued by the Office of the Inspector General highlighting the widespread "off-label use of atypical antipsychotic medication among nursing home residents, despite FDA warnings of increased risk of death when used to treat behavioral symptoms of distress in older adults with dementia." The initial overarching goal of this national partnership was to reduce the inappropriate use of antipsychotic drugs in long-stay nursing home residents through the use of person-centered, nonpharmacological interventions as the front-line approach to managing behavioral symptoms of dementia. At the start of the national partnership, Louisiana ranked 50th in the nation for the use of antipsychotics in long-stay residents, with a statewide prevalence of 29.7%.

To gain an understanding of factors that were contributing to this high use, Dr Spurlock was instrumental in the design of a survey to collect statewide data from nursing home staff on the perceived barriers to the reduction in the use of antipsychotics, perceived reasons for the initiation and/or the continued use of antipsychotics, and knowledge of person-centered nonpharmacological interventions. Nurses also responded to specific items on the survey that assessed their knowledge regarding the potential adverse effects of antipsychotics in older adults.

Based on findings from the survey, barriers that identified were lack of knowledge of nondrug interventions to manage behavioral symptoms of dementia, and the lack of physician and family support to reduce antipsychotic medications. Using the findings from the survey, Dr Spurlock led efforts to tailor a statewide educational outreach aimed to reduce the use of antipsychotics in Louisiana's nursing homes. Dr Spurlock's main role was to educate nursing home staff on person-centered, nonpharmacological interventions as the front-line approach in managing behavioral and psychological symptoms of dementia. This was accomplished in workshops conducted across the state and attended by staff representing 150 different nursing homes. On-site training was also conducted at nursing homes with the highest use of antipsychotics. This on-site strategy increased the participation of direct care staff, such as certified nursing assistants, who provide the most direct care for residents. In addition, nurses attended an educational session: "Antipsychotic Medications and Older Adults: What Every Nurse Should Know." Content included information on the impact of normal age-related physiologic changes on pharmacokinetics, side effects of antipsychotics, inappropriate behavioral target symptoms for use of antipsychotics (ie, wandering and resistance to care), and evaluation of the resident's response to antipsychotic medications based on target symptoms. Additional resources were also shared with the staff such as the American Geriatrics Society *Beers Criteria for Potentially Inappropriate Medication Use in Older Adults*.[34]

Success in reducing the use of antipsychotic medications in nursing homes also requires the support of family members/consumers. To garner their support, Dr Spurlock planned and conducted educational sessions in public places (ie, conference rooms in libraries) on nonpharmacological approaches and potential dangers in using antipsychotics to treat behavioral symptoms of dementia. Finally, she engaged consultant pharmacists and prescribers of antipsychotics, including physicians and advanced practice nurses. Existing tools such as the Minimum Data Set (MDS), the Certification and Survey Provider Enhanced Reporting (CASPER), and the consultant pharmacist reports were used as pragmatic measures for tracking potentially inappropriate use of antipsychotics.

The official measure of the National Partnership is the percentage of long-stay residents who are receiving an antipsychotic medication, excluding those with diagnoses of schizophrenia, Huntington's Disease, or Tourette's Syndrome. According to the most recent CMS quarterly prevalence report on antipsychotic use for long-stay residents (2020 quarter 2), 15.4% of Louisiana's long-stay residents were receiving an antipsychotic medication, a significant decrease from the initial 29.7%. Although gains have been made, on-going interdisciplinary collaboration and regular monitoring through a continuous quality improvement process are necessary to continue this positive trend. More importantly, the reduction in antipsychotic medications contributes to positive resident, clinician, and family outcomes such as improved quality of life for residents with dementia, an improved work environment for the clinicians, and enhanced family satisfaction.

Gaps in Care for Older Adults in Long-Term Care

Dementia, depression, delirium, and anxiety disorders are the most prevalent psychiatric disorders among older adults in long-term care.[35] Despite the plethora of regulations governing long-term care facilities, there are still gaps and room for improvement in caring for older adults in nursing homes with significant mental health disorders. Geropsychiatric nurses can help bridge these gaps.

Gaps in clinical care include the limited evidence base on the efficacy of nonphar-macological interventions for neuropsychiatric symptoms such as sleep disturbances and aggression, and insufficient evidence on the effectiveness, side effects, and inter-actions of psychoactive and other medications. Older adults often have a higher prev-alence of comorbid chronic health conditions, in addition to psychiatric disorders. Multiple comorbid health conditions add to the risk of overprescribing, drug interac-tions, and treatment complications. While regulatory pressures have reduced the use of psychotropic medications in nursing homes, the absence of a strong evidence base underlying other medications for older adults, who are often frail and have mul-tiple comorbid health conditions, is disturbing. This problem is especially evident for medications used off-label, such as some antidepressants. Even when medications are prescribed for therapeutic purposes rather than for chemical restraint, possible toxicities and dangerous interactions may be underestimated. Identifying the potential for aggression (before it occurs) in older adults in nursing homes with a diagnosis of dementia and effectively managing aggressive symptoms remains a crucial challenge. Aggression poses a danger to other vulnerable older adults in the nursing home and caregivers. Better ways to identify triggers and defuse them are urgently needed.

The COVID-19 pandemic has created unique challenges and opportunities for ger-opsychiatric nurses at the bedside, those in nursing home leadership, and advanced practice nurses. One of the COVID-19-related challenges is new or worsening mental health symptoms. Many older adults, families, caregivers, and providers experienced mental health consequences, such as depression, anxiety, grief, and fear during the pandemic, and these consequences may linger. Current evidence indicates resur-gence in cases as social distancing restrictions were lifted. Evidence is needed on how to best preserve and protect the short- and long-term well-being of older adult residents, families, caregivers, and providers. Although the pandemic continues to negatively affect the well-being of many, social distancing restrictions have positively influenced the adoption of telehealth and other technologies in long-term care. Addi-tional data are needed to better understand the efficacy, adoption, and costs of providing geropsychiatric care using different technologies.[36]

CLINICAL RESEARCH PRIORITIES

The authors recognize that there are many clinical research studies needed to address gaps in care for older adults residing in long-term care who have mental health disor-ders. While the scope of this article prevents an exhaustive list, we present several pri-orities for future research.

1. Where we do have sufficient evidence, conduct embedded pragmatic trials to enhance the uptake of EBP (see Collaborative Care of Depression IMPACT trial)[37]
2. Determine how to promote social interaction while balancing safety with respect to infection control
3. Develop and test person-centered outcomes that matter to older adults living with mental health problems (see Alzheimer's Association practice guidelines)[38]
4. Rigorous, adequately powered, placebo-controlled, randomized, double-blind controlled clinical trials are needed to determine the most effective nonpharmaco-logical interventions for sleep, agitation, aggression, and other common neuropsy-chiatric symptoms.[38]
5. Existing large databases and new databases should be created to analyze the effectiveness, side effects, and interactions of medications commonly prescribed for older long-term care residents. These studies should be adequately powered to examine multiple correlations.

6. Determine how best to mitigate the short and long-term mental health effects of the 2020 to 21 COVID-19 pandemic and the ongoing resurgence. Outcomes of importance include the mental health of residents, families, caregivers, and providers, and the economic impact on nursing homes.

7. As the demands for providing complex GPN care and improving business efficiency in nursing home settings increase, rigorous experimental research evaluating the efficacy, adoption, and costs of telemedicine (synchronized video communications between a provider and a patient) and telehealth (video conferencing, remote patient monitoring, store and forward technologies, and mobile health applications) is needed. Telemedicine and telehealth may help address the lack of on-site expertise and communication challenges.

8. Assess the psychometric properties of aggression scales in diverse populations, and to develop and validate instruments that predict aggression. Almost all (96%) persons with dementia display severe aggression at least once during their illness.[38]

As previous surveys[8–10] have shown, there is minimal education provided across the curriculum in GPN neither at the baccalaureate level nor advanced practice level. One of the important outcomes from the Geropsychiatric Nurse Collaborative was the development of GPN competencies across nursing curriculums particularly in advanced practice nursing. These recommended competencies are freely available on the Portal of Geriatric Online Education (www.Pogoe.com/).[2] Stephens and colleagues[39] provided a robust list of educational and practice resources for GPN (p. 282). There is also an effort underway to develop a certificate recognition through GAPNA for the top of the APRN pyramid.[40] The top of the pyramid is focused on specialty certifications, typically identified and provided by professional organizations. These recognitions are focused on a health care need.[40] Expertise in geropsychiatric advanced practice nursing fits well within the top of the pyramid.

SUMMARY

GPN leaders have the expertise to address common psychiatric conditions in long-term care settings, from ADRD, anxiety, depression, delirium, and delirium superimposed on dementia to substance misuse issues and serious mental illnesses including bipolar disorders, schizophrenia, and schizoaffective disorder. Expertise in evidence-based medication and nonpharmacological treatments of these disorders is an expectation of geropsychiatric nurses. Consultation with and education of colleagues on the evidence-based interventions is provided by GPN leaders in long-term care to improve interprofessional care.

Professional organizations are recognizing the importance of GPN. The Geropsychiatric Nursing Collaborative is an extension of the work started by Drs Evans, Beck, and Buckwalter initially housed with the American Academy of Nursing and funded through the John A. Hartford Foundation[2,3] The Geropsychiatric Nurse Collaborative is currently a special interest group within the National Hartford Center of Gerontological Nursing Excellence.[39] In addition, GAPNA has a very active special interest group in GPN. As mentioned earlier members of this special interest group published a position paper supporting GPN as a subspecialty of gerontological advanced practice nursing. The American Psychiatric Nursing Association frequently features professional speakers on geropsychiatric topics. Interprofessional groups also engage advanced practice nurses. The formally named organization the American Medical Directors Association (AMDA), now called AMDA - The Society for Post-Acute and Long-Term Care Medicine, includes advanced practice nurses working in long-term care.

Many of these APRNs are focused on GPN. AMDA recently started a Behavioral Health Work Group to address the mental health issues in long-term and postacute care.[41] The American Association of Geriatric Psychiatry also has an advanced practice nurses' caucus for their APRNs in GPN. As you might imagine, geropsychiatric nurses belong and engage with several of these professional organizations to advance their knowledge and the knowledge of others in GPN leadership.

GPN leaders address essential health care needs from dementia to substance misuse and serious mental illness. Developing new evidence and/or using evidence-based interventions to improve the lives of older adults with psychiatric conditions is rewarding work. We welcome any and all nurses interested to become GPN leaders.

CLINICS CARE POINTS

- Nurses specializing in multiple disciplines contribute to the care of persons living with dementia.

- Person-centered, evidence based, nonpharmacological interventions are first line approaches for the treatment of behavioral and psychological symptoms of dementia.

- Off label use of atypical antipsychotic medications in persons with dementia continue despite FDA warnings of increased risk of stroke or death in persons with dementia.

- A survey in long-term care, found that barriers to reducing antipsychotic medications included lack of knowledge of nonpharmacological interventions and lack of physican and family support to reduce antipsychotic medications.

- Regular monitoring of antipsychotic medication use through continuous quality improvement is necessary to reduce the use of antipsychotic medications and improve the quality of life for nursing home residents with dementia.

- Nursing home residents suffer from multiple chronic conditions increasing the risk of polypharmacy and adverse drug events.

ACKNOWLEDGMENTS

Pamela Cacchione acknowledges the Jonas Foundation Vision Scholars Program.

DISCLOSURE

The authors have nothing to disclose.

REFERENCES

1. American Academy of Nursing, Hartford Geriatric Nursing Initiative, and John A. Hartford Foundation. Geropsychiatric Nursing Collaborative work group: Definition of geropsychiatric nursing. 2010. Available at: https://pogoe.org/sites/default/files/Definition_Ger-opsych_Nursing.pdf. Accessed November 7, 2020.

2. Beck C, Buckwalter K, Evans L. Geropsychiatric nursing competency enhancements. definition of geropsychiatric nursing portal of geriatric online education. 2012. Available at: https://pogoe.org/sites/default/files/Definition_Geropsych_Nursing.pdf. Accessed 7/2/2021.

3. American Academy of Nursing. Geropsychiatric nursing collaborative. 2021. Available at: https://www.aannet.org/initiatives/early-initiatives/geropsychiatric-nursing-collaborative. Accessed 7/2/2021.

4. Chong TWH, Curran E, Ames D, et al. Mental health of older adults during the COVID-19 pandemic: lessons from history to guide our future. Int Psychogeriatr 2020;32(10):1249–50.
5. Institute of Medicine. The mental health and substance use workforce for older adults. In: Whose hands? Washington, DC: National Academies Press; 2012.
6. A. Stecker. An oral history of Dr. Mary Starke Harper 2021. Available at: https://www.youtube.com/watch?v=mi30GSAkaaA. Accessed April 16, 2021.
7. Morris DL, Mentes J. Geropsychiatric nursing education: challenge and opportunity. J Am Psychiatr Nurses Assoc 2006;12(2):105–15.
8. Evans LK, Buckwalter KC. Geropsychiatric nursing. timing is everything, and this is the time. [Editorial]. J Am Psychiatr Nurses Assoc 2006;12:74.
9. Geropsychiatric Nurse Collaborative. Geropsychiatric nursing: state of the future conference. J Am Psychiatr Nurses Assoc 2006;12(2–3).
10. Kolanowski A, Piven ML. Geropsychiatric nursing: the state of science. J Am Psych Nurs Assoc 2006;12(2):75–99.
11. Stolley JM, Buckwalter KC, Harper MS. Unity in diversity. Outcomes of the Geropsychiatric nursing survey. J Psychosoc Nurs Ment Health Serv 1994;32(12):35–9. PMID: 7714851.
12. Kurlowicz LH, Puentes WJ, Evans LK, et al. Graduate education in geropsychiatric nursing: Findings from a national survey. Nurs Outlook 2007;55:303–10.
13. Stephens C, Harris M, Buron B. The current state of U.S. geropsychiatric graduate nursing education: Results of the national geropsychiatric graduate nursing education survey. J Am Psychiatr Nurs Assoc 2015;21(6):385–94.
14. Harris M, Buron W, Stephens C. Embracing the challenges in graduate geropsychiatric nursing. J Prof Nurs 2018;34(3):221–5.
15. Beck C, Buckwalter KC, Dudzick PM, et al. Filling the void in geriatric mental health: the geropsychiatric nursing collaborative as a model for change. Nurs Outl 2011;59(4):236–41. https://doi.org/10.1016/j.outlook.2011.05.016.
16. Stephens C, Evans LK, Bradway C, et al. Challenges in aging, dementia and mental health: New knowledge and energy to inform solutions. J Am Geriatr Soc 2018;66(suppl 1):S1–3.
17. Journal of the American Geriatrics Society. Special Issue: State of the Future in Global Aging, Dementia and Mental Health: Bridging Leadership in Science, Practice, Education and Policy. 2018;66 (Suppl 1):S1–S57.
18. Puentes WJ, Buckwalter K, Evans LK. Geropsychiatric nursing: Planning for the future. J Am Psychiatr Nurses Assoc 2006;12(3):165–9.
19. Harris M, Devereaux Melillo K, Keilman L, et al. *GAPNA Position Statement:* supporting evidence for geropsychiatric nursing as a subspecialty of gerontological advanced practice nursing. Geriatr Nurs 2021;42(1):247–50.
20. American Nurses Association. Gerontological nursing: scope and standards of gerontological nursing practice. Silver Springs, MD: Author; 2019.
21. American Psychiatric Association. Diagnostic and statistical manual of mental disorder. 5th ed. Arlington, VA: American Psychiatric Publishing; 2019.
22. Center for Disease Control and Prevention. What is dementia? 2021. Available at: https://www.cdc.gov/aging/dementia/index.html. Accessed June 29, 2021.
23. Harris-Kojetin L, Sengupta M, Lendon JP, et al. Long-term care providers and services users in the United States, 2015–2016. Nat Cent Hlth Stat Vit Hlth Stat 2019; 3(43):2019.
24. Kolanowski A, Cortes TA, Mueller C, et al. A call to the CMS: Mandate adequate professional nurse staffing in nursing homes. Am J Nurs 2021;121(3):22–5.

25. Harris M, Mayo A, Balas M, et al. Trends and opportunities in geropsychiatric nursing: Enhancing practice through specialization and interprofessional education. J Nurs Ed 2013;52(6):317–21.
26. Harrington C, Carrillo H, Garfield R, et al. KFF. Nursing facilities, staffing, residents and facility deficiencies, 2009 through 2016. 2018. Available at: https://files.kff.org/attachment/REPORT-Nursing-Facilities-Staffing-Residents-and-Facility-Deficiencies-2009-2016; https://www.cms.gov/Medicare/Provider-Enrollment-and-Certification/CertificationandComplianc/Downloads/nursinghomedata compendium_508-2015.pdf. Centers for Medicare and Medicaid Services. Nursing home data compendium 2015 edition.
27. Perez-Ros P, Martinez-Arnau FM, Baixauli-Alacreu S, et al. Delirium predisposing and triggering factors in nursing home residents: a cohort trial-nested case-control study. J Alzheimers Dis 2019;70:1113–22.
28. Administration on Aging, Administration for Community Living profile of older Americans, 2018. US Department of Health and Human Services. Available at: https://acl.gov/sites/default/files/Aging%20and%20Disability%20in%20America/2017OlderAmericansProfile.pdf. Accessed 2017.
29. Grabowski D, Aschbrenner K, Rome V, et al. Quality of mental health care for nursing home residents: A literature review. Med Care Res Rev 2010;67(6):627–56. Available at: https://www.ncbi.nlm.nih.gov/pmc/articles/PMC2981653/pdf/nihms-203623.pdf. Accessed July 1, 2021.
30. Shippee TP, Weiwen NG, Bowblis JR. Does living in a higher proportion minority facility improve quality of life for racial/ethnic minority residents in nursing homes? Innovation in Aging 2020;4(3):igaa014.
31. Kolanowski A, Van Haitsma K. Nursing Home Toolkit. Promoting positive behavioral health. (n.d.) Available at: http://www.nursinghometoolkit.com/. Accessed May 20, 2021.
32. Mueller C, Bowers B, Burger S, et al. American Academy of Nursing on policy. Policy brief: Registered nurse staffing requirements in nursing homes. Nurs Outl 2016;64:507–9.
33. CMS.gov [Internet]. Baltimore (MD); Centers for Medicare and Medicaid Services. Press release, CMS announces partnership to improve dementia care in nursing homes 2012. Available at: https://www.cms.gov/newsroom/press-releases/cms-announces-partnership-improve-dementia-care-nursing-homes. Accessed June 14, 2021.
34. American Geriatrics Society. Updated AGS Beers criteria for potentially inappropriate medication use in older adults. J Am Geriatr Soc 2019;67(4):674–94. https://doi.org/10.1111/jgs.15767.
35. Seitz D, Purandare N, Conn D, et al. Prevalence of psychiatric disorders among older adults in long-term care homes: A systematic review. Int Psychoger 2010;22(7):1025–39. https://doi.org/10.1017/S1041610210000608.
36. Seitz DP, Brisbin S, Herrmann N, et al. Efficacy and feasibility of nonpharmacological interventions for neuropsychiatric symptoms of dementia in long term care: a systematic review. JAMDA 2012;13(6):503–6. https://doi.org/10.1016/j.jamda.2011.12.059.
37. Hunkeler EM, Katon W, Tang L, et al. Long term outcomes from the IMPACT randomized trial for depressed elderly patients in primary care. BMJ 2006;332(7536):259–63. https://doi.1136/bmj.38683.710255.BE.
38. Alzheimer's Association. Dementia care practice recommendations. Available at: https://www.alz.org/professionals/professional-providers/dementia_care_practice_recomendations. Accessed on 9/20/2021.

39. Stephens C, Massimo L, Harris M, et al. Advances in geropsychiatric nursing: a decade in review. Arch Psychiatr Nurs 2020;34(5):P281–7. https://doi.org/10.1016/j.apnu.2020.07006.

40. National council of state boards of nursing Consensus model of APRN regulation: licensure, accreditation, Certification & Education 2008. Available at: https://www.ncsbn.org/Consensus_Model_for_APRN_Regulation_July_2008.pdf. Accessed April 19, 2021.

41. AMDA the society for post-acute and long-term care medicine. Committees 2021. Available at: https://paltc.org/committees?_ga=2.242979266.1957064959.1629151479-1366787152.1629151479. Accessed July 26, 2021.

The Advanced Practice Registered Nurse Leadership Role in Nursing Homes
Leading Efforts Toward High Quality and Safe Care

Deb Bakerjian, PhD, APRN, FAAN, FAANP, FGSA,

KEYWORDS

- Nurse practitioners • Clinical nurse specialists • APRNs • Leadership
- Nursing homes • Skilled nursing facilities • Long-term care

KEY POINTS

- APRNs are knowledgeable and skilled in the care of older adults.
- There is abundant evidence that APRNs in nursing homes improve resident outcomes.
- The literature strongly supports that APRN leadership is needed and that policies must be revised to enable APRNs to lead in nursing homes.

INTRODUCTION/HISTORY/DEFINITIONS/BACKGROUND

This article provides evidence for the critical role of advanced practice registered nurse (APRN) leadership in the care of older adults living in the nursing home (NH). The older adult population in the NH is one of the frailest, marginalized, and often neglected in American society. Looking back at the impact of the COVID-19 pandemic on older adult NH residents reveals a stunning number of infections and subsequent deaths in long-term care facilities (659,617 confirmed resident cases and 133,443 confirmed deaths as of July 11, 2021).[1] This is a shameful reminder of the many challenges and gaps in the long-term care industry including inadequate staffing, high staff turnover, improper isolation technique, and lack of fundamental knowledge of how to adequately implement infection control and prevention processes.[2]

Long-term care includes a wide variety of health care facilities outside of acute care hospitals that offer different levels of care, depending on the needs of the patients. Skilled nursing facilities or NHs provide postacute and long-term care to patients and residents that includes 24-hour skilled nursing care and regular visits by physicians and advanced practice providers and are the focus of this article.

Betty Irene Moore School of Nursing at UC Davis, 2570 48th Street, Sacramento, CA 95817, USA
E-mail address: dbakerjian@UCDAVIS.EDU
Twitter: @DebBakerjian (D.B.)

Nurs Clin N Am 57 (2022) 245–258
https://doi.org/10.1016/j.cnur.2022.02.011
0029-6465/22/© 2022 Elsevier Inc. All rights reserved.
nursing.theclinics.com

There are four core roles for APRNs in the United States: nurse practitioner (NP), clinical nurse specialist (CNS), certified nurse-midwife, and certified registered nurse anesthetist.[3] APRN practice scope and standards vary by state and are governed primarily by the individual state boards of registered nursing. NPs and CNSs are certified based on the APRN consensus model, which addressed the regulatory inconsistencies in the United States; identified the four core APRN roles; and further delineated six population foci including family, adult-gerontology, neonatal, pediatrics, women's health/gender-related, and psychiatric-mental health.[4] Long-term care settings primarily involve family, adult-gerontology, and psychiatric-mental health foci; however, there are pediatric long-term care facilities as well.

NPs and CNS have some core clinical roles and responsibilities in common; however, there are some differences in their education, licensure, and practice. NPs are autonomous and collaborative in their approach to care. The main role of the NP in the NH is to improve access to care by providing direct clinical care to individual patients.[5,6] In this role, they assess residents, order diagnostic tests, diagnose, order treatments, prescribe medications, and perform procedures within their scope of practice. NPs provide care to long-stay residents overall, for acute exacerbations of chronic conditions, and for residents with neuropsychiatric (dementia, depression, anxiety) diagnoses when compared with physicians.[7] The quality of NP care is similar to, or in some cases better, than that of physicians in several studies.[8–13]

CNSs in NH have often acted more in a consulting role to the organization to improve overall quality of care versus providing individual care to residents.[14,15] CNSs focus on guiding the overall management of the frail, complex older adult population, educating and supporting the NH staff to provide optimal care using the best available evidence, and facilitate a supportive culture of safety in the organization. This role has been driven by research and quality improvement efforts, led by CNSs with gerontologic expertise.[14,16]

Over the years there have been increasing questions about how to differentiate the roles of NPs and CNSs with some studies finding confusion, ambiguity, and lack of clarity in the two roles.[17,18] Some authors have advocated for the blending or combining the role of NPs and CNSs indicating the roles have more in common than differences,[19–21] whereas others have supported that the roles are distinct and should remain as two separate, important roles that address different needs.[22,23]

COMPETENCIES

NPs and CNSs core competencies include a similar focus of expertise in direct patient care, education, research, ethical, and leadership. However, there are several differences. NP competencies in the care of older adults are driven by National Organization of Nurse Practitioner Faculties and include nine broad categories of competence:[24]

1. Scientific foundations
2. Leadership
3. Quality
4. Practice inquiry
5. Technology and information literacy
6. Policy
7. Health delivery system
8. Ethics
9. Independent practice

In addition, the competencies are further delineated along populations, with family and adult-gerontologic primary care NPs having competencies in the care of older adults. CNS competencies in the care of older adults include[25]

1. Direct care
2. Consultation
3. Systems leadership
4. Collaboration
5. Coaching
6. Research
7. Ethical decision-making, moral agency, and advocacy

To work in a primary care environment, CNSs can obtain a CNS core certification or an adult-gerontology CNS certification through the American Nurses Credentialing Center. Alternatively, they can also obtain certification as an adult-gerontologic acute care NP through the American Association of Critical Care Nurses.

An important area of commonality between NPs and CNSs is in leadership, and both professions have a stated core competency in leadership. The focus of leadership is slightly different.

NP leadership competencies are the same for family and adult-gerontology primary care NPs and include:

1. Assumes complex and advanced leadership roles to initiate and guide change.
2. Provides leadership to foster collaboration with multiple stakeholders (eg, patients, community, integrated health care teams, and policy makers) to improve health care.
3. Demonstrates leadership that uses critical and reflective thinking.
4. Advocates for improved access, quality, and cost-effective health care.
5. Advances practice through the development and implementation of innovations incorporating principles of change.
6. Communicates practice knowledge effectively, orally and in writing.
7. Participates in professional organizations and activities that influence advanced practice nursing and/or health outcomes of a population focus.

CNSs have a core set of leadership competencies that tend to focus more on health systems and populations. The competencies listed next are specific to adult-gerontology population primary care NPs because these are most relevant to NH care:

1. Integrates information technology into systems of care to enhance safety and monitor health outcomes.
2. Creates therapeutic health-promoting, aging-friendly environments.
3. Promotes health care policy and system changes that facilitate access to care and address biases.
4. Provides leadership to address threats to health care safety and quality in the adult–older adult population.
5. Participates in development, implementation, and evaluation of clinical practice guidelines that address patient needs across the adult age spectrum.
6. Advocates for access to hospice and palliative care services for patients across the adult age spectrum.
7. Promotes system-wide policies and protocols that address cultural, ethnic, spiritual, and intergenerational/age differences among patients, health care providers, and caregivers.
8. Implements system-level changes based on analysis and evaluation of age-specific outcomes of care.

This article focuses on the leadership role of NPs and CNSs in NH.

NURSE PRACTITIONERS AND CLINICAL NURSE SPECIALISTS LEADERSHIP IN NURSING HOMES

The complexity of care has expanded in NHs over the past few decades with the rise of postacute care discharges; in response, APRNs have developed five distinct roles in NHs including[5]

- Direct, ongoing primary care management for long-term care residents
- Acute care to short-stay patients and long-stay residents
- Education to staff, residents, and family members
- Consultation to NH staff on system-wide patient care clinical issues including care coordination, discharge planning, and care transitions
- Consultation to organizations on improving patient safety and quality systems within the facility

Based on the NP and CNS competencies, there are leadership responsibilities in each of these roles, with NPs having greater roles and responsibilities in providing individual care to NH residents[8,9,26] and CNSs carrying out more of the consulting role.[15,27,28] However, the literature shows that NPs have provided consultation to NH staff and organizations in areas of quality improvement and patient safety.[29–31] For example, geriatric NPs were used as consultants in education and quality improvement in the Wellspring project to improve the quality of care in 11 freestanding NHs.[32] Both NPs and CNSs work to improve patient safety and the quality of care for residents in NHs.

Leading in Patient Care

APRNs, particularly NPs at the patient care level, have assumed increasing responsibilities for leading the individual care of residents in NHs. Multiple studies have shown that NPs provide equivalent or better care in NHs, often at a lower cost.[8,9,26,29–31] From the perspective of APRN leadership in NHs, this may mean leading the clinical care teams working closely and collaborating with directors of nursing, directors of staff development, quality leaders, infection preventionists, and other clinical staff. NPs provide leadership when they engage staff in "on the spot" or "just in time" education.

One example of a best practice is to conduct rounds with the certified nursing assists (CNAs) and or charge nurses on patients, engage in discussion of specific patient care issues, and look for opportunities to reinforce knowledge, which has been shown to be highly successful in hospitals.[33] These are great opportunities to reinforce clinical issues, particularly related to areas that the CNA or licensed nurse are responsible for. For example, in the process of helping a CNA to turn a resident, the APRN can model examining the skin for rashes or signs of pressure injury and talk about what to look for or ask the staff what they would be looking for, always keeping the discussion on a positive note and commending staff for a job well done when appropriate. An opportunity with the staff nurse would be initiating walking rounds to review diagnoses, medications, and discuss whether medications and treatments are working as intended and look for any potential patient safety concerns. These leadership practices elevate the entire team in the NHs by extending knowledge and reinforcing competence and confidence in the staff.

CNSs do not typically provide direct resident care themselves, although that does happen in some cases. More importantly, CNSs can greatly influence the staff and how they interact with patients. For example, a best practice for the CNS could be to work with licensed nurses and certified nursing assistants to teach them how to do walking rounds at change of shift or rounding with the CNAs to assess for pain.[34,] These opportunities might include piloting rounds on a specific group of residents or by working with the nurses and CNAs to determine what data should be exchanged during walking rounds and end with conducting a class where the process is demonstrated with a simulated patient.

Advanced Practice Registered Nurse Leadership at the Organizational Level

One of the key messages in the 2011 Institute of Medicine (now National Academies of Medicine [NAM]) report: *The Future of Nursing: Leading Change, Advancing Health*[35] and the 2021 NAM report *The Future of Nursing 2020 to 2030: Charting a Path to Achieve Health Equity*[42] is that nurses, in partnership with other health professionals, must be strong leaders to ensure a transformed health system. Specifically, the reports call on nurses to be full partners and to lead in the design, implementation, evaluation, and advocacy reforms in future health systems. This requires an even greater focus on strong nursing leadership at all levels within the profession of nursing and interprofessionally through collaborative efforts with other health professions. Nowhere is this more urgent than in NHs, were team-based care is essential.

There are many long-standing systems-level problems in NHs that should be addressed and APRNs certainly have the knowledge, skills, and ability to lead many of the reform efforts. These issues vary depending on the context, time, and perspective. In 2006, the Commonwealth Fund highlighted the booklet, *20 Common Nursing Home Problems—and How to Resolve Them* (https://www.commonwealthfund.org/publications/other-publication/2006/jan/twenty-common-nursing-home-problems-and-how-resolve-them). The 20 problems included such issues as resident rights and honoring resident preferences, but also clinical issues, such as appropriate use of medications, avoiding the use of restraints, minimizing the use of feeding tubes, frequent readmissions, and refusal of medical treatments.

In the past two decades, other significant areas of concern have included inadequate staffing,[36–38] excessive antipsychotic use,[39] high staff turnover,[40] and poor NH culture.[41] In response to the many quality issues, Centers for Medicare and Medicaid Services (CMS) launched a demonstration project on quality assurance performance improvement (QAPI) as an outgrowth of the Affordable Care Act. QAPI integrates two components of quality: quality assurance ensures that minimum standards are met, and performance or quality improvement focuses on constant improvement processes. APRNs have been shown to be natural leaders of these efforts.

More recently, the issue of institutional racism has been identified as a key national and health system problem. The NAM recently published *The Future of Nursing 2020 to 2030: Charting a Path to Achieve Health Equity*, which provides a framework for how nurses can see their role in acknowledging and addressing the significant challenges in health and health care and the impact on patients.[42] The report included nine recommendations for system-wide changes to support nurses in their work to positively influence health equity. Disparities in US NHs have existed for many years, Feng and colleagues[43] reported on the growth of people of color in NHs because of the increased growth of older minority populations. Rahman and Foster[44] found that families of color preferences for NHs that are close to family and with racial homogeneity foster racial segregation in communities of color and contribute to disparities in quality. Despite this knowledge, little has been done to address these disparities.[43–48] In fact, a 2015 study of Medicare and Medicaid dual eligible residents identified quality disparities between access to CMS publicly reported five-star NHs and

NHs with lower quality ratings. In 2020, the COVID-19 pandemic revealed significant racial and ethnic disparities with greater numbers of residents of color becoming infected and dying from the disease. In one study, NHs with higher numbers of racial and ethnic minority residents had 61% more COVID-19-related deaths compared with NHs without racial and ethnic minorities.[46] APRNs are well positioned to lead the work of reducing disparities in NHs by devising and leading quality improvement projects that address deficiencies and areas of low quality as identified in CMS NH Compare Web site.

Advanced Practice Registered Nurse Leading Quality Improvement

In the first decade of the twenty-first century, there were a variety of studies examining APRNs leading quality improvement in NHs that revealed higher quality in homes with APRN consultant leaders compared with NHs that lack the APRN consultant.[14,49–51] Using an APRN, whether a consultant or an employee, has consistently shown positive outcomes through APRN-led quality improvement projects.

Building on the positive outcomes of early quality improvement efforts, the Advancing Excellence in America's Nursing Homes campaign, which is now known as the National Nursing Home Quality Improvement initiative, formed in 2007 to enhance quality improvement in NHs at a national level.[51] The original Advancing Excellence campaign focused on an interdisciplinary group of national leaders coming to consensus on a set of quality measures that encouraged participating NHs to set achievement goals and submit measures over time. APRNs held several leadership positions in the campaign and were key participants in this process.[52] The campaign relied on local area networks of excellence to create learning collaboratives to assist NHs to establish goals and processes and to enter data in a national database.[53] The campaign was active for several years and provided a strong foundation for the subsequent work on the QAPI process.

The QAPI framework involves five elements: (1) design and scope; (2) governance and leadership; (3) feedback, data systems, and monitoring; (4) performance improvement projects; and (5) systematic analysis and systemic action and requires multiple steps to implement.[54] The complexity of the process has been challenging at times for some NHs to initiate and sustain,[55,56] partially because of minimal nurse leader staff. Registered nurse leaders including the director of nursing and APRNs have been essential in the successful implementation of QAPI in NHs,[57] particularly those with gerontologic nursing knowledge who can lead the interdisciplinary team.[52] Early studies of QAPI implementation revealed that many NHs were not ready to implement QAPI; they lacked skills needed to identify, measure, and remedy deficiencies in the NH.[58] APRN Leaders can gain from the lessons learned from the Advancing Excellence Campaign and from QAPI implementation to use their leadership skills and knowledge of the quality improvement process to assist NHs to implement QAPI programs.

A Quality Improvement Leadership Exemplar

One of the most informative studies of the leadership role of APRNs in improving NH care came from the Missouri Quality Improvement Initiative (MOQI) study where APRNs working full time were embedded in 16 NHs; the study aimed to reduce potentially avoidable hospital transfers from NHs to acute care hospitals.[59] The role of the APRNs (15 NPs and 1 CNS) was to work with the existing NH staff and leadership to manage sick residents and to affect changes in NH systems that would improve resident outcomes. The APRNs were supported by a variety of experts including an INTERACT/Quality Improvement coach, care transitions coach, health informatics coordinator, MOQI medical director, and project supervisor along with the research team. APRNs kept diaries to document how they interacted in the home.

Based on the APRN notes, the key areas of impact include taking care of basics, such as improving hydration, mobility, preventing falls, and managing medications; improving team discussions about implementing comfort care and limiting treatments, such as advance directives, cardiopulmonary resuscitation orders, and hospice; and improving communication about treatments, such as counseling families, working with staff and families, and obtaining assistance from social work staff. APRNs used root cause analysis to help staff understand the causes of poor outcomes, initiated huddles to identify issues and develop solutions, and to affect changes in medications by reducing polypharmacy and ensuring best practices were followed. APRNs were instrumental in improving discussions about key issues in quality of care and in improving communication with residents and family. The MOQI project is an excellent exemplar in how APRNs can lead quality improvement and practice transformation in NHs.

A later report on this work showed statistically significant reductions in all-cause hospitalizations (40%; $P < .001$), avoidable hospitalizations (45.2%; $P < .001$), all-cause emergency department visits (50.2%; $P < .001$), and in avoidable emergency department visits (59.7%; $P < .001$). Medicare costs were also reduced, as were outcome measures, such as falls, incontinence, and immobility.[59] The authors emphasized that the APRN primary focus was on the geriatric clinical management of residents. APRNs emphasized the importance of discontinuing harmful or ineffective care and instead to focus on evidence-based practices and held direct care staff accountable for their care processes.

Findings include that there are essential elements in the APRN role in the areas of leadership, direct resident care, and education including:

- Leadership: APRNs must lead and advocate for evidence-based practices and be part of the facility leadership team
- Direct resident care: early recognition of changes of condition and management of acute and chronic illness
- Education: educate staff, residents, and family on goals of care, health management, and planning for end-of-life care

These three areas are competencies for NPs and CNSs. These reports also acknowledge the importance of the context and tools that enabled the success of the APRNs in this project including the use of the INTERACT II (https://pathway-interact.com/) tools, such as Stop and Watch and SBAR (situation, background, assessment, recommendation). When the leadership remained engaged and the APRNs were supported in this work, the improvements were sustained over time.[60]

Advanced Practice Registered Nurses Improving Nursing Home Outcomes

Several studies have shown that APRNs can reduce the cost of care and improve important resident outcomes, such as resident satisfaction, emergency room visits, and hospitalizations.[8,61–63] In a 2005 systematic review, Christian and Baker[11] found that when NPs were part of the team, there were lower rates of emergency department transfer and shorter hospital lengths of stay. A later study using Medicare claims data found that NP visits were associated with fewer emergency department visits overall and fewer hospitalizations when compared with physician-only visits.[64] APRNs are instrumental in improving a variety of other quality outcomes, such as resident falls, urinary incontinence, depression, pressure injuries, and behaviors.[51,65]

Another successful role for APRNs is in improving NH outcomes through the change management process. In a study of NPs and CNSs as change champions in implementing an evidence-based pain protocol, Kaasalainen and colleagues[34] reported that APRNs used multiple strategies to promote changes in pain management including education of team members, staff reminders highlighting the pain protocol, chart audits, feedback, staff meetings, NPs using advanced assessment skills, and other quality improvement initiatives. By using interactive educational meetings and encouraging the entire interdisciplinary team to participate in discussions around the pain protocol, staff were empowered to initiate practice changes. The study authors conclude that APRNs can improve the quality of care in NHs by leading staff through knowledge transfer and exchange to achieve positive outcomes.[34]

A third major way in which APRNs have shown significant success is in leading transitions of care, where APRNs facilitate care as patients leave the acute care setting and transition to other settings including NHs. A major goal of Mary Naylor's transitional care model is to reduce rehospitalizations in vulnerable populations including older adults. The transitional care model used APRNs because they are uniquely qualified to work with other members of the interdisciplinary team on complex issues, such as medication reconciliation, geriatric syndromes, and management of high-risk residents.[66,67] The transitional care model includes such processes as engaging the resident and caregiver, managing symptoms, educating residents, promoting self-management, collaborating with the team, coordinating care, and maintaining relationships; practices that APRNs are already skilled at providing in NHs.[68]

There are two other models that are applicable to NHs. The first is the GRACE model (geriatric resources for assessment and care of elders), which is focused on care of older adults with care provided primarily by a NP and social worker who collaborate with an expanded GRACE team that includes a geriatrician, geriatric pharmacist, physical therapist, and mental health case worker.[69] This is an integrated care model that targets mostly dual-eligible (Medicare and Medicaid) patients with chronic diseases. Care begins with a comprehensive in-home assessment by an NP and social worker, who then consult with the expanded team. A randomized controlled trial that studied the model found that patients enrolled in GRACE had fewer emergency room visits, hospitalizations, readmissions, and lower costs compared with a control group.[70,71] This is particularly effective in caring for older adults with multiple chronic diseases and mental health and psychosocial challenges. Many of these patients have conditions that are well managed by nurses, such as common geriatric syndromes including pressure ulcers, incontinence, and functional decline. This model is highly effective during transitions of care.

The second model is the NICHE-LTC (Nurses Improving Care for Healthsystem Elders-Long-Term Care) program. This program is an education and consultation model with the aim to improve health care at the organizational level. Key components of the program include the geriatric resource nurse along with the geriatric certified nursing assistant, who work together as champions for frontline staff as organizations work to implement evidence-based processes into the workflow.[71] APRNs often play an important role in leading this program in NHs with goals of improving mobility, reducing falls, preventing avoidable emergency department visits and hospitalizations, preventing pressure injuries, and other resident outcomes.

BARRIERS TO ADVANCED PRACTICE REGISTERED NURSE LEADERSHIP

There are several organizational barriers to the ability of APRNs to impact quality outcomes. A recent systematic review identified facilitators to an optimal practice environment, which included an autonomous/independent practice environment and positive relationships with physicians.[72] Organizational barriers included poor physician and administrator relationships, a lack of understanding of the APRN role, along with various policy and regulatory barriers to practice. The authors stress that organizations must explain and promote the APRN role, implement policies that support APRNs, and communicate these with members of the organization to ensure a positive practice environment.

The most prominent barriers to APRN leadership are the disjointed scope of practice regulations in the United States,[73] inconsistent and confusing insurance practices, and the consistent opposition of the American Medical Association,[74] who insist that increased scope of practice is a patient safety risk, despite all evidence to the contrary.[75] As discussed throughout this article, there are many studies that have shown that NP care is safe, results in similar outcomes to physicians, at lower cost, and often with greater patient and family satisfaction. One of the most relevant studies was undertaken by the Institute of Medicine Report in 2010.

The 2011 Institute of Medicine Report, *The Future of Nursing: Leading Change, Advancing Health*, called for removing practice barriers for APRNs as one of their key messages.[35] Subsequently, other national organizations have published statements of agreement with these recommendations. The National Governors Association published their own review of the evidence, advocating for expanded use of APRNs and for states to consider changing their scope of practice restrictions.[76] The Robert Wood Johnson Foundation published a comprehensive overview of the scope of practice and other regulatory barriers to APRN practice in *Charting Nursing's Future*, which discusses misconceptions, barriers to APRN practice, recent breakthroughs, and remaining barriers.[77] The report can be downloaded from the Web site at https://www.rwjf.org/en/library/research/2017/03/the-case-for-removing-barriers-to-aprn-practice.html. This report makes a strong case for removing these barriers to APRN practice.

The newest NAM report, *The Future of Nursing 2020 to 2030: Charting a Path to Achieve Health Equity*,[42] reinforces the need for APRN full scope of practice in Recommendation 4: all organizations, including state and federal entities and employing organizations, should enable nurses to practice to the full extent of their education and training by removing barriers that prevent them from more fully addressing social needs and social determinants of health and improving health care access, quality, and value. These barriers include regulatory and public and private payment limitations; restrictive policies and practices; and other legal, professional, and commercial (contracts and customary practices) impediments.

OPPORTUNITIES FOR ADVANCED PRACTICE REGISTERED NURSE LEADERS IN POLICY CHANGE

Gutchell and colleagues[78] discuss the rationale and best practices for removing practice barriers through health policy changes using Kingdon's theoretic framework of agenda setting and emphasize the importance of taking advantage of the window of opportunity that arises when a problem, policy, and political streams come together to create an opportunity for policy change. The authors describe various strategies that are effective in changing health care policies related to APRN scope of practice. Some of these strategies are understanding the political climate, coalition building, choosing an influential sponsor, conducting letter writing campaigns, meeting with and developing relationships with legislators and staff, raising public awareness, and developing fact sheets, among other activities.

SUMMARY

There is strong evidence that APRNs provide high-quality care in NHs and that they play an important leadership role at many levels. At the individual care level as clinicians, APRNs lead the clinical care of residents and engage with NH staff to improve individual resident quality of care that results in improved resident outcomes. They also play an important role in leading resident, family, and staff education and facilitate communication among the team.

At the organization of system level, APRNs act as consultants and lead QAPI efforts. In this role, they lead teams of staff to work together to set goals, implement improvement processes, measure the improvements, and put systems in place to reinforce and sustain improvements. They use their skills in communication, coordination, collaboration, and education to work with the staff to achieve the established goals.

There are barriers to APRN practice that interfere with optimization of these efforts. APRNs must use their leadership skills to reduce these barriers. APRN leadership efforts should initiate the published evidence-based practices as a call to action to address the various barriers to APRN scope of practice so that additional progress is made in improving the care of older adults in the NH setting. It is clear that there is more than enough evidence to support the need for APRN leadership; it is critical that APRNs use this evidence and their leadership to influence NH owners, operators, and policy makers to strengthen the APRN role in long-term care.

CLINICS CARE POINTS

- APRNs bring advanced clinical knowledge to nursing homes that improves patient outcomes.
- APRN leadership enhances nursing home processes of clinical care, which also contibute to improved resident care.
- Nursing homes should be mandated to hire APRNs to achieve improved resident outcomes, improve resident and staff satisfaction, and improve patient safety.

DISCLOSURE

The author has nothing to disclose.

REFERENCES

1. Data.CMS.gov. COVID-19 nursing home data. Available at: https://data.cms.gov/covid-19/covid-19-nursing-home-data. Accessed July 11, 2021.
2. Bakerjian D. Coronavirus disease 2019 (COVID-19) and safety of older adults. Agency for Healthcare Research and Quality Patient Safety Network. Available at: https://psnet.ahrq.gov/index.php/primer/coronavirus-disease-2019-covid-19-and-safety-older-adults#. Accessed July 11, 2021.
3. National Council on State Boards of Nursing (NCSBN). PRNS in the U.S. Available at: https://www.ncsbn.org/aprn.htm. Accessed July 11, 2022.
4. Stanley JM, Werner KE, Apple K. Positioning advanced practice registered nurses for health care reform: consensus on APRN regulation. J Prof Nurs 2009;25(6):340–8.
5. Bakerjian D. Care of nursing home residents by advanced practice nurses: a review of the literature. Res Gerontol Nurs 2008;1(3):177–85.

6. Bakerjian D. Nurse practitioners and primary care for older adults. In: Primary care for older adults. Cham: Springer; 2018. p. 159–72.

7. Bakerjian D, Harrington C. Factors associated with the use of advanced practice nurses/physician assistants in a fee-for-service nursing home practice: a comparison with primary care physicians. Res Gerontol Nurs 2012;5(3):163–73.

8. Stanik-Hutt J, Newhouse RP, White KM, et al. The quality and effectiveness of care provided by nurse practitioners. J Nurse Pract 2013;9(8):492–500.

9. Oliver GM, Pennington L, Revelle S, et al. Impact of nurse practitioners on health outcomes of Medicare and Medicaid patients. Nurs Outlook 2014;62(6):440–7.

10. Bauer JC. Nurse practitioners as an underutilized resource for health reform: evidence-based demonstrations of cost-effectiveness. J Am Acad Nurse Pract 2010;22(4):228–31.

11. Christian R, Baker K. Effectiveness of nurse practitioners in nursing homes: a systematic review. JBI Evid Synth 2009;7(30):1333–52.

12. Aigner MJ, Drew S, Phipps J. A comparative study of nursing home resident outcomes between care provided by nurse practitioners/physicians versus physicians only. J Am Med Dir Assoc 2004;5(1):16–23.

13. Kane RL, Garrard J, Skay CL, et al. Effects of a geriatric nurse practitioner on process and outcome of nursing home care. Am J Public Health 1989;79(9):1271–7.

14. Krichbaum KE, Pearson V, Hanscom J. Better care in nursing homes: advanced practice nurses' strategies for improving staff use of protocols. Clin Nurse Spec 2000;14(1):40–6.

15. Popejoy LL, Rantz MJ, Conn V, et al. Improving quality of care in nursing facilities: Gerontological clinical nurse specialist as research nurse consultant. Journal of Gerontological Nursing 2000;26(4):6–9.

16. Rantz MJ, Popejoy L, Petroski GF, et al. Randomized clinical trial of a quality improvement intervention in nursing homes. Gerontologist 2001;41(4):525–38.

17. Carter N. Clinical nurse specialists and nurse practitioners: title confusion and lack of role clarity. Nursing Leadership 2010;23:189–210.

18. Ormond-Walshe SE, Newham RA. Comparing and contrasting the clinical nurse specialist and the advanced nurse practitioner roles. J Nurs Manag 2001;9(4): 205–7.

19. Dudley-Brown S. Revisiting the blended role of the advanced practice nurse. Gastroenterol Nurs 2006;29(3):249–50.

20. Lynch AM. At the crossroads: we must blend the CNS+ NP roles. Online J Issues Nurs 1996;2(1).

21. Elder RG, Bullough B. Nurse practitioners and clinical nurse specialists: are the roles merging? Clin Nurse Spec 1990;4(2):78–84.

22. Mick DJ, Ackerman MH. Deconstructing the myth of the advanced practice blended role: support for role divergence. Heart Lung 2002;31(6):393–8.

23. Page NE, Arena DM. Rethinking the merger of the clinical nurse specialist and the nurse practitioner roles. Image J Nurs Sch 1994;26(4):315–8.

24. National Organization of Nurse Practitioner Faculties. Adult-gerontology acute care and primary care NP competencies.. Available at: https://cdn.ymaws.com/www.nonpf.org/resource/resmgr/files/np_competencies_2.pdf. Accessed July 11, 2021.

25. American Association of Colleges of Nursing. Adult-gerontology clinical nurse specialist competencies. Available at: https://nacns.org/wp-content/uploads/2016/11/adultgeroCNScomp.pdf. Accessed July 11, 2021.

26. Intrator O, Miller EA, Gadbois E, et al. Trends in nurse practitioner and physician assistant practice in nursing homes, 2000–2010. Health Serv Res 2015;50(6): 1772–86.

27. Mahler A. The clinical nurse specialist role in developing a geropalliative model of care. Clin Nurse Specialist 2010;24(1):18–23.

28. Naylor MD, Brooten D. The roles and functions of clinical nurse specialists. Image J Nurs Sch 1993;25(1):73–8.

29. Horner JK, Hanson LC, Wood D, et al. Using quality improvement to address pain management practices in nursing homes. J Pain Symptom Manage 2005;30(3): 271–7.

30. Ouslander JG, Lamb G, Tappen R, et al. Interventions to reduce hospitalizations from nursing homes: evaluation of the INTERACT II collaborative quality improvement project. J Am Geriatr Soc 2011;59(4):745–53.

31. Hanson LC, Reynolds KS, Henderson M, et al. A quality improvement intervention to increase palliative care in nursing homes. J Palliat Med 2005;8(3):576–84.

32. Stone RI, Reinhard SC, Bowers B, et al. Evaluation of the Wellspring model for improving nursing home quality. New York: Commonwealth Fund; 2002.

33. Sunkara PR, Islam T, Bose A, et al. Impact of structured interdisciplinary bedside rounding on patient outcomes at a large academic health centre. BMJ Qual Saf 2020;29(7):569–75.

34. Kaasalainen S, Ploeg J, Donald F, et al. Positioning clinical nurse specialists and nurse practitioners as change champions to implement a pain protocol in long-term care. Pain Manag Nurs 2015;16(2):78–88.

35. Shalala D, Bolton LB, Bleich MR, et al. The future of nursing: Leading change, advancing health. Washington DC: The National Academy Press; 2011. Available at: https://www.nap.edu/catalog/12956/the-future-of-nursing-leading-change-advancing-health. Accessed July 11, 2021.

36. Harrington C, Schnelle JF, McGregor M, et al. Article commentary: the need for higher minimum staffing standards in US nursing homes. Health Serv Insights 2016;9. HSI-S38994.

37. Harrington C, Dellefield ME, Halifax E, et al. Appropriate nurse staffing levels for US nursing homes. Health Serv Insights 2020;13. 1178632920934785.

38. Dellefield ME. The relationship between nurse staffing in nursing homes and quality indicators. J Gerontol Nurs 2000;26(6):14–28.

39. Gurwitz JH, Bonner A, Berwick DM. Reducing excessive use of antipsychotic agents in nursing homes. JAMA 2017;318(2):118–9.

40. Gandhi A, Yu H, Grabowski DC. High nursing staff turnover in nursing homes offers important quality information: study examines high turnover of nursing staff at US nursing homes. Health Aff 2021;40(3):384–91.

41. Grabowski DC, O'Malley AJ, Afendulis CC, et al. Culture change and nursing home quality of care. Gerontologist 2014;54(Suppl_1):S35–45.

42. Wakefield MK, Williams DR, Le Menestrel S, et al. The future of nursing 2020-2030: charting a path to achieve health equity. National Academies Press; 2021. Retrieved July 2021 fromAvailable at: https://nam.edu/publications/the-future-of-nursing-2020-2030. Accessed 2021.

43. Feng Z, Fennell ML, Tyler DA, et al. Growth of racial and ethnic minorities in US nursing homes driven by demographics and possible disparities in options. Health Aff 2011;30(7):1358–65.

44. Rahman M, Foster AD. Racial segregation and quality of care disparity in US nursing homes. J Health Econ 2015;39:1–16.

45. Tamara Konetzka R, Grabowski DC, Perraillon MC, et al. Nursing home 5-star rating system exacerbates disparities in quality, by payer source. Health Aff 2015; 34(5):819–27.
46. Weech-Maldonado R, Lord J, Davlyatov, et al. High-minority nursing homes disproportionately affected by COVID-19 Deaths. Front Public Health 2021;9:246.
47. Li Y, Cen X, Cai X, et al. Racial and ethnic disparities in COVID-19 infections and deaths across US nursing homes. J Am Geriatr Soc 2020;68(11):2454–61.
48. Sugg MM, Spaulding TJ, Lane SJ, et al. Mapping community-level determinants of COVID-19 transmission in nursing homes: a multi-scale approach. Sci Total Environ 2021;752:141946.
49. Rantz MJ, Vogelsmeier A, Manion P, et al. Statewide strategy to improve quality of care in nursing facilities. Gerontologist 2003;43:248–58.
50. Ryden MB, Snyder M, Gross CR, et al. Value-added outcomes: the use of advanced practice nurses in long-term care facilities. Gerontologist 2000;40: 654–62.
51. Healthcare Quality Improvement Campaign (n.d.). Advancing HealthCare Excellence Quality Campaigns. Available at: https://nhqualitycampaign.org/. Accessed July 11, 2021.
52. Bakerjian D, Beverly C, Burger SG, et al. Gerontological nursing leadership in the advancing excellence campaign: moving interdisciplinary collaboration forward. Geriatr Nurs 2014;35(6):417–22.
53. Bakerjian D, Bonner A, Benner C, et al. Reducing perceived barriers to nursing homes data entry in the Advancing Excellence Campaign: the role of LANEs (Local Area Networks for Excellence). J Am Med Directors Assoc 2011;12(7): 508–17.
54. CMS. QAPI resources. 2020. Available at: https://www.cms.gov/Medicare/Provider-Enrollment-and-certification/QAPI/qapiresources. Accessed July 11, 2021.
55. Bonner A. Hope springs eternal: can project echo transform nursing homes? J Am Med Directors Assoc 2021;22(2):225.
56. Unroe KT, Ouslander JG, Saliba D. Nursing home regulations redefined: implications for providers. J Am Geriatr Soc 2018;66(1):191–4.
57. Bakerjian D, Zisberg A. Applying the advancing excellence in America's nursing homes circle of success to improving and sustaining quality. Geriatr Nurs 2013; 34(5):402–11.
58. Smith KM, Castle NG, Hyer K. Implementation of quality assurance and performance improvement programs in nursing homes: a brief report. J Am Med Directors Assoc 2013;14(1):60–1.
59. Popejoy L, Vogelsmeier A, Galambos C, et al. The APRN role in changing nursing home quality: the Missouri quality improvement initiative. J Nurs Care Qual 2017; 32(3):196–201.
60. Vogelsmeier A, Popejoy L, Galambos C, et al. Results of the Missouri quality initiative in sustaining changes in nursing home care: six-year trends of reducing hospitalizations of nursing home residents. J Nutr Health Aging 2021;25(1):5–12.
61. Kane RL, Keckhafer G, Flood S, et al. The effect of Evercare on hospital use. J Am Geriatr Soc 2003;51(10):1427–34.
62. Buchanan JL, Bell RM, Arnold SB, et al. Assessing cost effects of nursing-home-based geriatric nurse practitioners. Health Care Financ Rev 1990;11(3):67.
63. Kane RL, Flood S, Keckhafer G, et al. Nursing home residents covered by Medicare risk contracts: early findings from the EverCare evaluation project. J Am Geriatr Soc 2002;50(4):719–27.

64. Bakerjian D, Dharmar M. Impact of nurse practitioner care of nursing home residents on emergency room use and hospitalizations. Innovation Aging 2017;703.
65. Capezuti E, Taylor J, Brown H, et al. Challenges to implementing an APN-facilitated falls management program in long-term care. Appl Nurs Res 2007; 20(1):2–9.
66. Naylor MD, Sochalski JA. Scaling up: bringing the transitional care model into the mainstream. Issue Brief (Commonw Fund) 2010;103(11):1–2.
67. Naylor MD, Hirschman KB, Toles MP, et al. Adaptations of the evidence-based transitional care model in the US. Soc Sci Med 2018;213:28–36.
68. Naylor MD. A decade of transitional care research with vulnerable elders. J Cardiovasc Nurs 2000;14(3):1–4.
69. AHRQ (n.d.). GRACE Team Care. Available at: https://www.ahrq.gov/workingforquality/priorities-in-action/grace-team-care.html. Accessed July 11, 2021.
70. Counsell SR, Callahan CM, Buttar AB, et al. Geriatric Resources for Assessment and Care of Elders (GRACE): a new model of primary care for low-income seniors. J Am Geriatr Soc 2006;54(7):1136–41.
71. NICHE Program (n.d.). NICHE Long-Term Care/NYU Rory Meyers College of Nursing. Available at: https://nicheprogram.org/sites/niche/files/inline-files/LTC_overview_2019_v041819_DIGITAL.pdf. Accessed July 11, 2021.
72. Schirle L, Norful AA, Rudner N, et al. Organizational facilitators and barriers to optimal APRN practice: an integrative review. Health Care Manage Rev 2020; 45(4):311–20.
73. AANP. Scope of practice for nurse practitioners. Available at: https://www.aanp.org/advocacy/advocacy-resource/position-statements/scope-of-practice-for-nurse-practitioners. Accessed July 11, 2021.
74. AMA. AMA successfully fights scope of practice expansions that threaten patient safety. Available at: https://www.ama-assn.org/practice-management/scope-practice/ama-successfully-fights-scope-practice-expansions-threaten. Accessed July 11, 2021.
75. Hain D, Fleck L. Barriers to nurse practitioner practice that impact healthcare redesign. Online J Issues Nurs 2014;19(2).
76. National Governors Association. The role of nurse practitioners in meeting increasing demand for primary care. Available at: https://www.nga.org/wp-content/uploads/2019/08/1212NursePractitionersPaper.pdf. Accessed July 11, 2021.
77. Fauteux N, Brand R, Fink JL, et al. The case for removing barriers to APRN practice. Charting Nursing's Future 2017;30:1–2.
78. Gutchell V, Idzik S, Lazear J. An evidence-based path to removing APRN practice barriers. J Nurse Pract 2014;10(4):255–61.

Nursing Leadership and Palliative Care in Long-Term Care for Residents with Advanced Dementia

Ruth Palan Lopez, PhD, GNP-BC, FGSA, FAAN[a],
Alison E. Kris, PhD, RN, FGSA[b],*,
Sarah C. Rossmassler, DNP, AGPCNP-BC, ANP-BC, ACHPN[a]

KEYWORDS

- Palliative care • Nursing home • Dementia • End-of-life care

KEY POINTS

- Many people with end-stage dementia receive care in nursing homes.
- Many nursing home residents experience uncomfortable interventions with little clinical benefit at the end of life, rather than palliative strategies aimed at achieving comfort.
- Nurses at all levels of practice are ideal providers to lead change in the delivery of palliative care to nursing home residents with advanced dementia.

INTRODUCTION

Alzheimer disease and related dementias (ADRD) are terminal conditions causing irreversible, progressive brain disorders that destroy memory, thinking, and eventually the ability to care for oneself. Worldwide, an estimated 47 million people are living with dementia; this figure is projected to increase to 66 million by 2030 and 115 million by 2050.[1] ADRD affects nearly 6 million people in the United States and is the fifth leading cause of death in people aged 65 and older.[2] Currently, there are no known treatments to prevent or stop the progression of the disease. In the final stage of the disease, advanced dementia, people have profound memory loss and are completely dependent in all activities of daily living. For those with advanced dementia, palliative care may offer a better quality of life than continued aggressive, burdensome interventions lacking significant clinical benefit.

[a] MGH Institute of Health Professions School of Nursing, 36 First Avenue, Boston, MA 02129, USA; [b] Marion Peckham Egan School of Nursing, Fairfield University, 1073 North Benson Road, Fairfield, CT 06824, USA
* Corresponding author.
E-mail address: akris@fairfield.edu

Nurs Clin N Am 57 (2022) 259–271
https://doi.org/10.1016/j.cnur.2022.02.006
0029-6465/22/© 2022 Elsevier Inc. All rights reserved.

Palliative care is care for people living with serious illness, which focuses on providing relief of physical symptoms and psychological and spiritual distress and is focused on maximizing quality of life. The purpose of this article is to raise awareness of the palliative care needs of nursing home (NH) residents with advanced dementia. The authors present emerging models of palliative care delivery and call on nurse leaders to step up and lead in long-term care to increase the likelihood that residents with dementia and their families receive high-quality care at the end of life.

Spanning a trajectory of approximately 10 years, ADRD frequently progresses through a series of stages ranging from mild to severe impairment in the domains of cognition and function. The final stage, also called advanced dementia, consists of profound memory deficits, minimal verbal communication, inability to ambulate, incontinence, and complete dependence in activities of daily living. The CASCADE (Choices, Attitudes, and Strategies for Care of Advanced Dementia at the End-of-Life) was a landmark study characterizing the terminal phase of ADRD. The investigators followed 323 NH residents with advanced dementia over an 18-month period and found that more than half (54.8%) of residents died. A large percentage of residents suffered from pneumonia (46.7%), febrile episodes (44.5%), and eating problems (85.8%), which are among the most common distressing symptoms in advanced dementia. These residents also suffered from distressing symptoms, such as dyspnea (46.7%) and pain (39.1%).[3–5] Advanced dementia is now recognized as the terminal phase of the disease with a similar symptom burden and prognosis as advanced cancer, and a palliative approach to care is recommended.[6]

Palliative care is the "active holistic care of individuals across all ages with serious health-related suffering due to severe illness and especially of those near the end of life. It aims to improve the quality of life of patients, their families and their caregivers."[7(p755)] The underlying tenets include patient- and family-centered care, continuity of care across all health settings, interdisciplinary team collaboration, relief from suffering and distress, and equitable access. In 2014, the European Association for Palliative Care published a white paper defining palliative care for older adults with dementia. They used a Delphi approach, including 64 experts from 23 countries, and identified 11 domains and 57 recommendations to guide clinical practice, policy, and research for people with dementia (**Table 1**).

CURRENT STATE OF NURSING HOME CARE AND ADVANCED DEMENTIA

More than half (55.6%) of all deaths of people with dementia take place in NHs,[8] making NHs an important setting of end-of-life care for this population. Sadly, numerous studies find poor-quality end-of-life care in NHs.[9–13] Although 95.2% of proxies indicated that comfort was their primary goal of care,[9] many residents with advanced dementia experience potentially uncomfortable interventions that may not be aligned with the goal of achieving comfort.[14–16] Moreover, the experience of end-of-life care may be of lower quality for ethnic and racial minorities who experience less pain and symptom management, less hospice use, and more frequent hospitalizations.[17] The increased hospitalization rate increases physical and emotional distress for both NH residents and families and provides no clinical benefit at the end of life.

Tube feeding remains common in advanced dementia despite 20 years of research that fails to demonstrate a benefit[18–20] and numerous position statements advocating against their use.[21–24] Hospital transfers are also common at end of life for NH residents with advanced dementia. On average, NH residents with advance dementia experience 1.6 hospital transfers in the last 90 days of life.[16] In a 5-year period (2011–2016), nearly half of all NH residents with advanced dementia experienced at

Table 1
Domains and recommendations of palliative care

NCP Domain	Recommendations
Domain 1: Structure and processes of care	Comprehensive interdisciplinary assessment of patient and family Addresses identified and expressed needs of patient and family Interdisciplinary team consistent with plan of care Education and training Emotional impact of work Team has relationship with hospices Physical environment meets needs of patient and family
Domain 2: Physical aspects of care	Pain, other symptoms, and treatment side effects are managed using best practices Team documents and communicates treatment alternatives permitting patient/family to make informed choices Family is educated and supported to provide safe/appropriate comfort measures to patient
Domain 3: Psychological and psychiatric aspects of care	Psychological and psychiatric issues are assessed and managed Team uses pharmacologic, nonpharmacologic, and complementary therapies as appropriate Grief and bereavement program is available to patients and families
Domain 4: Social aspects of care	Interdisciplinary social assessment Care plan developed Referral to appropriate services
Domain 5: Spiritual, religious, and existential aspects of care	Assesses and addresses spiritual concerns Recognizes and respects religious beliefs, provides religious support Makes connections with community and spiritual/religious groups or individuals as desired by patients/family
Domain 6: Cultural aspects of care	Assesses and aims to meet culture-specific needs of patients and families Respects and accommodates range of language, dietary, habitual, and ritual, practices of patients and families Team has access to/uses translation resources Recruitment and hiring practices reflect cultural diversity of community
Domain 7: Care of the imminently dying patient	Signs and symptoms of impending death are recognized and communicated As patient declines, team introduces or reintroduces hospice Signs/symptoms of approaching death are developmentally age and culturally appropriate

(continued on next page)

Table 1 (continued)	
NCP Domain	**Recommendations**
Domain 8: Ethical and legal aspects of care	Patient's goals, preferences, and choices are respected and form basis for plan of care Team is aware of and addresses complex ethical issues Team is knowledgeable about relevant federal and state statutes regulations

Copied with permission: Ferrell, B., Connor, S. R., Cordes, A., Dahlin, C. M., Fine, P. G., Hutton, N., ... & National Consensus Project for Quality Palliative Care Task Force Members. (2007). The national agenda for quality palliative care: The National Consensus Project and the National Quality Forum. *Journal of pain and symptom management, 33*(6), 737-744.

least one hospital transfer.[25] Reasons for these transfers are complex; however, they can include a lack of communication about goals of care, care inconsistent with what can be provided in an NH, and incomplete or uniformed advanced directives.[26] Hospitalization can be traumatic for NH residents with dementia, can lead to aggressive interventions, and are costly for the health care system. In addition, many older adults with dementia experience frequent transfers between hospital and NHs near the end of life.[16] They also undergo intensive rehabilitation. A study of 647 NHs in New York State found that 13.6% of long-stay decedent NH residents had therapy in the last month of life,[27] with many (16%) of them having very-high-intensity therapy (>500 hours) before death. A phenomenon Flint and colleagues[28(p2398)] termed "rehabbed to death," they point out that NHs are incentivized to provide curative and rehabilitation services rather than a palliative approach to care because Medicare pays for skilled services and NHs receive higher payments for those who received the most aggressive rehabilitation services.

PALLIATIVE CARE DELIVERY MODELS

Nursing leadership is required to transform palliative care within NHs in order to transform the current state of palliative care, using new models of care Kaasalainen and colleagues[29] identified 4 models of palliative care delivery in NHs: (1) external specialist end-of-life care model; (2) in-house end-of-life care; (3) in-house capacity building within a palliative care approach; and (4) in-house capacity building with external support from palliative specialist.

The External Specialist Model

In this model of care, NH residents who are considered near the end of life are referred to an external specialist team, and care is provided by this team.[29] An example of this model is hospice. To access hospice services in the NH setting, the resident's proxy must agree to forego curative treatment, and the resident's primary provider must certify that the resident has a short time to live, often less than 6 months. This transition to hospice care is often led by the charge nurse in the NH, who is the most involved with day-to-day care within NHs. The hospice team is led by a hospice registered nurse (RN), with consultation by a hospice physician, management of pain and other symptoms, education of NH staff and families, and provision of emotional and spiritual support for the resident and family. The NH charge nurse remains responsible for communicating and coordinating care with hospice, routine daily care, normally scheduled medical care, and medication and supplies not related to the resident's terminal illness. NH charge nurses are unique in that they retain primary responsibility as the center of coordination for hospice care in this setting. Since 1983, Medicare covers the cost of hospice but does not cover the cost of room and board, which remains the responsibility of the resident or, for those without funds, Medicaid.

Residents enrolled in hospice had fewer hospitalizations in the last 30 days of life,[30,31] were more likely to be assessed and treated for pain, were less likely to be restrained, have feeding tubes, intravenous or intramuscular injections, or have dyspnea compared with similar residents not enrolled in hospice.[32–35] In addition, family members reported higher perceptions of the quality of care and quality of dying.[36] However, hospice is still not widely used among dying NH residents and those with advanced dementia or used very late in the disease trajectory.[37]

There are also wide regional and racial differences.[38] Black residents compared with white residents have less favorable beliefs about hospice,[39] are less likely to use hospice,[17] and are more likely to revoke hospice to pursue life-prolonging therapies.[40] Accessing hospice is predominantly dependent on NH staff's ability and willingness to identify residents who may benefit; typically the charge nurse is the one leading this transition to hospice. Some family and staff consider hospice a form of giving up; there are gaps in the reimbursement system, and some NH believe that hospice is duplicative.[41]

In-House End-of-Life Care

In this model, care is provided in a special palliative care unit without relying on external specialists.[29] Nursing leadership within NHs would need to recognize the benefit of designing specialized units for the benefit of their residents at the end of life and lead the creation of these unique spaces. Despite a large number of NH residents who would benefit from receiving palliative care, Miller and Han[42] found that only 27% of US NHs have special programs or trained staff. There is little research on palliative special care units in NHs; however, research suggests NHs with special dementia units are less likely to have inappropriate antipsychotics, physical restraints, pressure ulcers, feeding tubes, and hospitalizations.[43] However, it has been known for decades that the formation of specialized units in hospitals results in improved patient care.[44] Additional research is needed to examine the influence of special care units on palliative and end-of-life care.

In-House Capacity Building Within a Palliative Care Approach

In-house capacity building within a palliative care approach involves building skill within the NH to promote high-quality palliative care for all residents.[29] Capacity building may include developing leadership teams or providing education, training, or tools. A promising intervention involved teaching NH staff members to serve as a leadership team of palliative care planning coordinators (PCPC) to facilitate family conferences and train staff in person-centered palliative care.[45] They tested the intervention in a cluster randomized clinical trial over an 18-month period in 20 NHs in Australia. In the intervention NHs, the PCPC identified residents with advanced dementia likely to benefit from a case conference, organized and chaired the interdisciplinary conferences with family members, developed and oversaw palliative care plans, and trained staff in person-centered palliative care. The primary outcome was family-rated end-of-life care. Secondary outcomes included nurse-rated resident level outcomes, such as quality of life, and symptoms care and NH variables, such as staff attitudes, knowledge, and confidence in providing palliative care. The use of this nursing leadership model resulted in reduced mortality during the study period, making it underpowered to assess the primary outcomes. However, they did find that those in the intervention arm provided care more consistent with a palliative approach, more frequent pain assessment, proactive identification of symptoms, and more comfort-related medications, such as analgesics. The NH provides a unique environment for nurses to autonomously lead clinical care and symptom management at the end of life.

In-House Capacity Building with External Support from Palliative Specialist

In-house capacity building with external support from palliative specialist is a hybrid model that focuses on developing capacity within the NH but also draws on external palliative expertise and nurse leadership to provide guidance to NH staff.[29] An example of this model of care was tested in 12 NHs in Australia.[46] Monthly Palliative Care Needs Rounds, chaired by specialist palliative care staff (nurse practitioners and clinical nurse specialists) and included NH staff, were used to discuss and plan care for residents who were at risk of dying and had high symptom burden. They found that the intervention improved the quality of death and improved staff awareness and capability in supporting the resident near the end of life. Rates of advance care planning and appointment of medical power of attorney also increased after implementation of these nurse-led Palliative Care Needs Rounds.

OPPORTUNITIES FOR PROFESSIONAL NURSE LEADERS

There is an overlap between excellent nursing care and palliative care.[47] According to the American Nurses Association, the goal of nursing care is to "protect, promote, and optimize health; to prevent illness and injury; to alleviate suffering; and to advocate for all populations."[48] Nursing care and palliative care alike require holistic assessment and treatment of physical, emotional, and spiritual health. Thus, although challenges to attaining high-quality palliative care for NH residents with advanced dementia have been identified, scrutiny of the challenges highlights opportunities for professional nurses to lead change. Opportunities include advocating for healthy work environments with sufficient RN staffing, ensuring dementia and palliative care education for all NH staff, empowering nurses to engage in advance care planning with families, and changing the paradigm of care from "comfort measures only" to ADVANCED-Comfort Care. The term ADVANCED-Comfort Care shifts the paradigm from one in which care is being taken away or removed, to one in which more advanced and intensive services are needed in order to meet end-of-life care goals.

The need to drive these system-based changes within NHs speaks to the need for excellence in NH leadership. Indeed, expert care, supervision by RNs, and strong professional leadership[49] are necessary for high-quality outcomes. Furthermore, successful palliative care takes leadership support.[50] Although research on nursing leadership within the administrative ranks of NHs is scant, existing research points to the need for additional leadership development for nurses in administrative roles. The most effective nursing leaders exhibit a transformational leadership style, defined by a style that engages, motivates, and empowers staff to lead change.

Unfortunately, leadership within NHs tends to be dominated by passive-avoidant leadership styles, in which the administration fails to inspire staff to engage in needed organizational transformations.[51] This passive-avoidant leadership style is associated with a variety of negative outcomes, including poor staff effectiveness, burnout, and lack of well-being.[52]

The culture of leadership across NHs requires change to advocate for safe work setting and conditions that are conducive to quality health care. Transformation from passive-avoidant leadership to transformational leadership is needed to enhance nurses' moral agency, support professional nursing practice, and allow nurses to practice to their full potential. Given the anticipated shortfalls across all nursing professions, these changes are needed to make NHs a valued place to work.

Advocate for Healthy Work Environments with Sufficient Registered Nurse Staffing in Nursing Homes

The profession of nursing, collectively through professional organizations, should articulate the need for sufficient skilled professional staff in NHs to meet residents' and families' needs and healthy working environments for those working in NHs. Health policy leadership is needed to ensure NHs have the funding necessary to support high-quality, end-of-life care. Research has demonstrated that residents in NHs with higher-than-average overall staffing ratios, and higher-than-average RN hours per patient day have better resident outcomes. Importantly, RN to licensed practical nurse (LPN) ratio may be more important to support palliative care programming rather than the overall nurse staff ratio.[53]

Staffing ratios are driven by, and responsive to, policy decisions at the state and federal level. Policies can serve both to establish staffing minimums and to ensure that adequate funding is present to support those minimums, and nursing leaders who have knowledge of long-term care need to be driving policy decisions at the state and local level.

Advocate for Dementia and Palliative Care Education for all Nursing Home Staff

In addition to leadership opportunities for the administrators to lead NHs to make meaningful transformations, there are leadership opportunities among schools of nursing to better educate students to provide better end-of-life care for residents with dementia. For years, studies have documented the inadequate training and education among NH staff in this area.[54,55]

Front-line NH staff (RNs, LPNs, certified nursing assistants) as well as physicians and nurse practitioners need and want additional training and leadership roles in palliative care.[53,56] A national survey of nurse practitioners working in hospice and palliative care found that less than half reported being adequately prepared in their graduate education.[57] To address this issue, Ersek and colleagues[58] developed a comprehensive, four-class program called Palliative Care Education Resource Team to enhance ability of end-of-life ability for nursing assistants and licensed nurses working in NHs. The curriculum was delivered to 169 staff members from 44 NHs. They found a significant increase in knowledge, self-rated perceived effectiveness, and supervisors' ratings of effectiveness in providing end-of-life care. All graduate nurses should have competency and leadership training in dementia and palliative care by integrating this content into nursing curricula to ensure that the nursing workforce can address palliative care needs of people with dementia across all settings. Furthermore, nurse leaders within NHs should ensure that nurses receive continuing education and professional development in these areas over time.

Empower Nursing Home Staff to Engage in Advance Care Planning with Proxy Decision Makers

Research over the last decade provides key insights into the drivers of end-of-life care for NH residents with advanced dementia.[59–66] Most notably, this research suggests that family members' preferences are a major determinant in intensity of end-of-life care, that they strive to do what is best, but struggle with uncertainty and a lack of guidance from health professionals.

Nurses in NHs frequently have intimate knowledge of residents and trusting relationships with their families. However, some nurses do not have sufficient evidence-based information on care strategies for people with advanced dementia and do not feel empowered to engage in these discussions.[67,68] Therefore, empowering nurses with up-to-date information on palliative strategies for people with advanced dementia and skills in engaging in end-of-life conversations is critically important.

Change the Paradigm of Care from Comfort Measures Only to ADVANCED-Comfort

Advance care planning and appointing a surrogate decision maker are critically important for those with dementia to ensure that residents' preferences are documented and that care decisions are concordant with those goals.[69] Ideally, the process begins early, before people lose the ability to make their wishes known. Advance care planning should be viewed as an ongoing conversation with a skilled clinician that takes place regularly and with any change in residents' condition. However, advance care planning in NHs is frequently framed as a dichotomous choice between "doing everything" (eg, full code) or "comfort measures only" (eg, do-not-resuscitate).

However, the provision of palliative care for NH residents should not be dependent on code status, and end-of-life conversations should not be framed as a dichotomous choice between "prolonging life" or "achieving comfort." Instead, all residents with advanced dementia, regardless of code status, should be offered intensive individualized comfort care that aims to improve quality of life by ameliorating distressing physical symptoms, providing psychological and spiritual care, and supporting family members.[70]

Nurses should take the lead in ensuring that residents' needs are identified and that the interdisciplinary NH team partners with families to develop a comprehensive plan based on the best available evidence to address those needs. This care should be branded as ADVANCED-Comfort care, reimbursed as a skilled service, and made known that one does not need to "give up" or "let go" to be made comfortable. This philosophy rejects the notion that the end of life is a time when "nothing more can be done." Instead, palliative care embraces the idea that an intense focus on high-quality, physical, psychological, and spiritual care of residents and their families, centered on quality of life requires more comprehensive care that extends beyond curative goals, increased and more comprehensive interdisciplinary resources, and advanced education of staff.

SUMMARY

To achieve high-quality palliative care, integrated leadership will be needed across several domains of nursing practice. Educational leadership is needed to ensure the next generation of nurses is equipped with the knowledge and skills to provide high-quality nursing care. Systems leadership is needed to transform NHs to support nurses to transform facilities to make the structural changes needed to better implement best knowledge and practice. Policy leadership is needed at both state and federal levels to advocate for changes in Medicare and Medicaid funding to drive NHs to improve staffing levels and skill mix across all NHs and to promote equity in palliative care.

In NHs, nurses have historically taken leadership roles at the bedside, as partner disciplines are often less present in this environment. In addition to leadership at the bedside, leadership across the domains of administration, education, and policy, nursing needs to take an expanded leadership role in choreographing and coordinating the care delivered by the partner health professions that play an important role in holistic care at the end-of-life.[71] In order to support the changes needed to improve end-of-life care for these residents, we need to advocate for dementia and palliative care education, empower NH staff to engage in advance care planning, and shift the paradigm of care from comfort measures "Only" to ADVANCED-Comfort.

CLINICS CARE POINTS

- Nursing home residents with advanced dementia should receive high-quality care aimed at achieving comfort and quality of life.
- Interventions that have no clinical benefit, such as feeding tubes, should be avoided.
- Family members who serve as proxy decision makers should be included as partners in designing care for residents with advanced dementia.

DISCLOSURE

The authors have nothing to disclose.

REFERENCES

1. Livingston, et al. 2017.
2. Zhao L. Alzheimer's disease facts and figures. Alzheimers Dement 2020;16: 391–460.
3. Mitchell SL, Kiely DK, Hamel MB. Dying with advanced dementia in the nursing home. Arch Intern Med 2004;164(3):321–6. https://doi.org/10.1001/archinte.164.3.321.
4. Mitchell SL, Kiely DK, Jones RN, et al. Advanced dementia research in the nursing home: the CASCADE study. Alzheimer's Dis Assoc Disord 2006;20(3): 166–75.
5. Mitchell SL, Teno JM, Kiely DK, et al. The clinical course of advanced dementia. N Engl J Med 2009;361(16):1529–38. https://doi.org/10.1056/NEJMoa0902234.
6. Sampson EL. Palliative care for people with dementia. Br Med Bull 2010;96(1): 159–74.
7. Radbruch L, De Lima L, Knaul F, et al. Redefining palliative care—a new consensus-based definition. J Pain Symptom Manage 2020;60(4):754–64.
8. Xu W, Wu C, Fletcher J. Assessment of changes in place of death of older adults who died from dementia in the United States, 2000–2014: a time-series cross-sectional analysis. BMC Public Health 2020;20(1):765. https://doi.org/10.1186/s12889-020-08894-0.
9. Engel SE, Kiely DK, Mitchell SL. Satisfaction with end-of-life care for nursing home residents with advanced dementia. J Am Geriatr Soc 2006;54(10):1567–72.
10. Shield RR, Wetle T, Teno J, et al. Vigilant at the end of life: family advocacy in the nursing home. J Palliat Med 2010;13(5):573–9. https://doi.org/10.1089/jpm.2009.0398.
11. Teno JM, Gruneir A, Schwartz Z, et al. Association between advance directives and quality of end-of-life care: a national study. J Am Geriatr Soc 2007;55(2): 189–94. https://doi.org/10.1111/j.1532-5415.2007.01045.x.
12. Toles M, Song M-K, Lin F-C, et al. Perceptions of family decision-makers of nursing home residents with advanced dementia regarding the quality of communication around end-of-life care. J Am Med Directors Assoc 2018;19(10):879–83.
13. Wetle T, Shield R, Teno J, et al. Family perspectives on end-of- life care experiences in nursing homes. Gerontologist 2005;45(5):642–50. https://doi.org/10.1093/geront/45.5.642.

14. Fulton AT, Gozalo P, Mitchell SL, et al. Intensive care utilization among nursing home residents with advanced cognitive and severe functional impairment. J Palliat Med 2014;17(3):313–7. https://doi.org/10.1089/jpm.2013.0509.

15. Teno JM, Gozalo P, Khandelwal N, et al. Association of increasing use of mechanical ventilation among nursing home residents with advanced dementia and intensive care unit beds. J Am Med Assoc Intern Med 2016;176(12):1809–16. https://doi.org/10.1001/jamainternmed.2016.5964.

16. Teno JM, Mitchell SL, Skinner J, Kuo S, Fisher E, Intrator O. Churning: the association between health care transitions and feeding tube insertion for nursing home residents with advanced cognitive impairment. J Palliat Med 2009;12(4): 359–62.

17. Estrada LV, Agarwal M, Stone PW. Racial/ethnic disparities in nursing home end-of-life care: a systematic review. J Am Med Dir Assoc 2021;22(2):279–90.e271. https://doi.org/10.1016/j.jamda.2020.12.005.

18. Minaglia C, Giannotti C, Boccardi V, et al. Cachexia and advanced dementia. J Cachexia Sarcopenia Muscle 2019;10(2):263–77. https://doi.org/10.1002/jcsm.12380.

19. Sampson EL, Candy B, Jones L. Enteral tube feeding for older people with advanced dementia. Cochrane Database Syst Rev 2009;4.

20. Teno JM, Gozalo PL, Mitchell SL, et al. Does feeding tube insertion and its timing improve survival? J Am Geriatr Soc 2012;60(10):1918–21.

21. American Geriatrics Society Choosing Wisely Workgroup. American Geriatrics Society identifies five things that healthcare providers and patients should question. J Am Geriatr Soc 2013;61:622–33. https://doi.org/10.1111/jgs.12226.

22. American Geriatrics Society Ethics, C., Clinical, P., & Models of Care, C. American Geriatrics Society feeding tubes in advanced dementia position statement. J Am Geriatr Soc 2014;62(8):1590–3. https://doi.org/10.1111/jgs.12924.

23. Ayman AR, Khoury T, Cohen J, et al. PEG insertion in patients with dementia does not improve nutritional status and has worse outcomes as compared with PEG insertion for other indications. J Clin Gastroenterol 2017;51(5):417–20. https://doi.org/10.1097/mcg.0000000000000624.

24. Bentur N, Sternberg S, Shuldiner J, et al. Feeding tubes for older people with advanced dementia living in the community in Israel. Am J Alzheimers Dis Other Demen 2015;30(2):165–72. https://doi.org/10.1177/1533317514539726.

25. McCarthy EP, Ogarek JA, Loomer L, et al. Hospital transfer rates among US nursing home residents with advanced illness before and after initiatives to reduce hospitalizations. JAMA Intern Med 2020;180(3):385–94.

26. Ouslander JG, Lamb G, Perloe M, et al. Potentially avoidable hospitalizations of nursing home residents: frequency, causes, and costs. J Am Geriatr Soc 2010; 58(4):627–35.

27. Temkin-Greener H, Lee T, Caprio T, et al. Rehabilitation therapy for nursing home residents at the end-of-life. J Am Med Directors Assoc 2019;20(4):476, 480. e471.

28. Flint LA, David D, Lynn J, et al. Rehabbed to death: breaking the cycle. J Am Geriatr Soc 2019;67(11):2398–401.

29. Kaasalainen S, Sussman T, McCleary L, Thompson G, Hunter PV, Wickson-Griffiths A. Palliative care models in long-term care: a scoping review. Nurs Leadersh (Tor Ont) 2019;32(3):8–26. https://doi.org/10.12927/cjnl.2019.25975.

30. Cai S, Miller SC, Gozalo PL, Nursing home-hospice collaboration and end-of-life hospitalizations among dying nursing home residents. J Am Med Dir Assoc 2018; 19(5):439–43. https://doi.org/10.1016/j.jamda.2017.10.020.

31. Gozalo P, Plotzke M, Mor V, et al. Changes in Medicare costs with the growth of hospice care in nursing homes. N Engl J Med 2015;372(19):1823–31.

32. Gage B, Miller S, Mor V, et al. Synthesis and analysis of Medicare's hospice benefit. Executive summary and recommendations. Rep prepared Off Disabil Aging Long Term Care Pol Off Assistant Secretary Plann Eval 2000;1–20.

33. Givens JL, Lopez RP, Mazor KM, et al. Sources of stress for family members of nursing home residents with advanced dementia. Alzheimer's Dis Assoc Disord 2012;26(3):254–9. https://doi.org/10.1097/WAD.0b013e31823899e4.

34. Miller SC, Lima JC, Mitchell SL. Influence of hospice on nursing home residents with advanced dementia who received Medicare-skilled nursing facility care near the end of life. J Am Geriatr Soc 2012;60(11):2035–41.

35. Stevenson DG, Bramson JS. Hospice care in the nursing home setting: a review of the literature. J Pain Symptom Manage 2009;38(3):440–51.

36. Teno JM, Gozalo PL, Lee IC, et al. Does hospice improve quality of care for persons dying from dementia? J Am Geriatr Soc 2011;59(8):1531–6.

37. Epstein-Lubow G, Fulton AT, Marino LJ, et al. Hospice referral after inpatient psychiatric treatment of individuals with advanced dementia from a nursing home. Am J Hosp Palliat Med 2015;32(4):437–9. https://doi.org/10.1177/1049909114531160.

38. Wang S-Y, Aldridge MD, Gross CP, et al. End-of-life care intensity and hospice use: a regional-level analysis. Med Care 2016;54(7):672–8. https://doi.org/10.1097/MLR.0000000000000547.

39. Johnson KS, Kuchibhatla M, Tanis D, et al. Racial differences in hospice revocation to pursue aggressive care. Arch Intern Med 2008;168(2):218–24. https://doi.org/10.1001/archinternmed.2007.36.

40. Johnson KS, Kuchibhatla M, Tulsky JA. What explains racial differences in the use of advance directives and attitudes toward hospice care? J Am Geriatr Soc 2008;56(10):1953–8.

41. Rodriquez J, Boerner K. Social and organizational practices that influence hospice utilization in nursing homes. J Aging Stud 2018;46:76–81. https://doi.org/10.1016/j.jaging.2018.06.004.

42. Miller SC, Han B. End-of-life care in U.S. nursing homes: nursing homes with special programs and trained staff for hospice or palliative/end-of-life care. J Palliat Med 2008;11(6):866–77. https://doi.org/10.1089/jpm.2007.0278.

43. Joyce NR, McGuire TG, Bartels SJ, et al. The impact of dementia special care units on quality of care: an instrumental variables analysis. Health Serv Res 2018;53(5):3657–79.

44. Aiken L, Sloane D. Effects of specialization and client differentiation on the status of nurses: the case of AIDS. J Health Social Behav 1997;8(3):203–22. https://doi.org/10.2307/2955367.

45. Agar M, Luckett T, Luscombe G, Phillips J, Beattie E, Pond D, Brooks D. Effects of facilitated family case conferencing for advanced dementia: a cluster randomized clinical trial. PloS one 2017;12(8). e0181020.

46. Liu WM, Koerner J, Lam L, et al. Improved quality of death and dying in care homes: a palliative care stepped wedge randomized control trial in Australia. J Am Geriatr Soc 2020;68(2):305–12. https://doi.org/10.1111/jgs.16192.

47. Hagan TL, Xu J, Lopez RP, et al. Nursing's role in leading palliative care: a call to action. Nurse Educ Today 2018;61:216–9. https://doi.org/10.1016/j.nedt.2017.11.037.

48. White, K. M. (2012). The essential guide to nursing practice: Applying ANA's scope and standards to practice and education: American Nurses Association.

49. Kolanowski A, Cortes TA, Mueller C, Bowers B, Boltz M, Bakerjian D. A call to the CMS: mandate adequate professional nurse staffing in nursing homes. AJN The Am J Nurs 2021;121(3):24–7.

50. Cloutier D, Stajduhar KI, Roberts D, et al. 'Bare-bones' to 'silver linings': lessons on integrating a palliative approach to care in long-term care in Western Canada. BMC Health Serv Res 2021;21(1):610. https://doi.org/10.1186/s12913-021-06606-x.

51. Poels J, Verschueren M, Milisen K, et al. Leadership styles and leadership outcomes in nursing homes: a cross-sectional analysis. BMC Health Serv Res 2020;20:1–10. https://doi.org/10.1186/s12913-020-05854-7.

52. Cummings GG, Tate K, Lee S, et al. Leadership styles and outcome patterns for the nursing workforce and work environment: a systematic review. Int J Nurs Stud 2018;85:19–60.

53. Harrington C, Schnelle JF, McGregor M, Simmons SF. Article commentary: The need for higher minimum staffing standards in US nursing homes. Health services insights 2016;9.

54. Anstey S, Powell T, Coles B, et al. Education and training to enhance end-of-life care for nursing home staff: a systematic literature review. BMJ Support Palliat Care 2016;6:353–61.

55. Brazil K, Brink P, Kaasalainen S, et al. Knowledge and perceived competence among nurses caring for the dying in long-term care homes. Int J Palliat Nurs 2012;18:77–83.

56. Kamal AH, Wolf SP, Troy J, Leff V, Dahlin C, Rotella JD. Policy changes key to promoting sustainability and growth of the specialty palliative care workforce. Health Aff 2019;38(6):910–8.

57. Pawlow P, Dahlin C, Doherty CL, et al. The hospice and palliative care advanced practice registered nurse workforce: results of a national survey. J Hosp Palliat Nurs 2018;20(4):349–57.

58. Ersek M, Grant MM, Kraybill BM. Enhancing end-of-life care in nursing homes: Palliative Care Educational Resource Team (PERT) program. J Palliat Med 2005;8(3):556–66.

59. Lopez RP. Suffering and dying nursing home residents: nurses' perceptions of the role of family members. J Hosp Palliat Nurs 2007;9(3):141–9.

60. Lopez RP. Decision-making for acutely ill nursing home residents: nurses in the middle. J Adv Nurs 2009a;65(5):1001–9. https://doi.org/10.1111/j.1365-2648. 2008.04958.x.

61. Lopez RP. Doing what's best: decisions by families of acutely ill nursing home residents. West J Nurs Res 2009b;31(5):613–26.

62. Lopez RP, Amella EJ, Mitchell SL, et al. Nurses' perspectives on feeding decisions for nursing home residents with advanced dementia. J Clin Nurs 2010; 19(5–6):632–8. https://doi.org/10.1111/j.1365-2702.2009.03108.x.

63. Lopez RP, Guarino AJ. Uncertainty and decision making for residents with dementia. Clin Nurs Res 2011;20(3):228–40. https://doi.org/10.1177/1054773811405521.

64. Lopez RP, Guarino AJ. Psychometric evaluation of the surrogate decision making self-efficacy scale. Res gerontological Nurs 2013;6(1):71–6. https://doi.org/10.3928/19404921-20121203-02.

65. Lopez RP, Mazor KM, Mitchell SL, et al. What is family-centered care for nursing home residents with advanced dementia? Am J Alzheimer's Dis Other Demen 2013;28(8):763–8. https://doi.org/10.1177/1533317513504613.

66. Lopez RP, Mitchell SL, Givens JL. Preventing burdensome transitions of nursing home residents with advanced dementia: it's more than advance directives. J Palliat Med 2017;20(11):1205–9. https://doi.org/10.1089/jpm.2017.0050.

67. Lopez RP, Amella EJ. Intensive individualized comfort care: making the case. J gerontol Nurs 2012b;38(7):3–5.

68. Lopez RP, Amella EJ, Strumpf NE, et al. The influence of nursing home culture on the use of feeding tubes. Arch Intern Med 2010;170(1):83–8. https://doi.org/10.1001/archinternmed.2009.467.

69. Hanson LC, Zimmerman S, Song MK, et al. Effect of the goals of care intervention for advanced dementia: a randomized clinical trial. JAMA Intern Med 2017; 177(1):24–31. https://doi.org/10.1001/jamainternmed.2016.7031.

70. Lopez RP, Amella EJ. Intensive individualized comfort care: making the case. J Gerontol Nurs 2012;38(7):1–3.

71. National Academies of Sciences, Engineering, and Medicine. The future of nursing 2020–2030: charting a path to achieve health equity. Washington, DC: The National Academies Press; 2021. https://doi.org/10.17226/25982.

Social Isolation and Nursing Leadership in Long-Term Care: Moving Forward After COVID-19

Diana Lynn Woods, PhD, RN, APRN-BC, FGSA[a],*,
Adria E. Navarro, PhD, LCSW[b], Pamela LaBorde, DNP, APRN, CCNS[c],
Margaret Dawson, LCSW[d], Stacy Shipway, MSN, PHN, DNP(c)[e]

KEYWORDS

- Long-term care • Nursing leadership • Social isolation • Social engagement
- Residential care • Older adults

KEY POINTS

- Understand the importance of social engagement and connectedness is essential. Critical considerations include avoiding social isolation for those with dementia and planning for activities to increase social engagement for LTC residents.
- Nursing leadership is needed to foster open communication and strategies to prevent social isolation and foster an inclusive environment to build a healthy community.
- Interdisciplinary programs that nurture engagement and connectedness are essential to prevent resident decline and meet the cultural, functional, spiritual, and social needs.
- Collaboration among professional disciplines, nursing, social work, rehabilitation services, medicine, and chaplaincy cannot be overemphasized.
- If/when quarantine is required, plan for continued social engagement and connectedness among residents.

INTRODUCTION

The 2020 to 2021 COVID-19 pandemic shed light on a longstanding problem in long-term care (LTC), the need for nursing leadership compounded by a heightened awareness of the impact of social isolation. Implementing the coronavirus precautions demanded by the pandemic resulted in the unintended consequences of social isolation for many residents, especially those vulnerable individuals with dementia. Moreover, increased

[a] Department of Doctoral Programs, School of Nursing, Azusa Pacific University, 701 East Foothill Boulevard, Building 1, Azusa, CA 91702-7000, USA; [b] Department of Social Work, Azusa Pacific University, 901 East Alosta Avenue, Azusa, CA 91702, USA; [c] University of Arkansas for Medical Sciences College of Nursing, 4301 West Markham, Slot 526, Little Rock, AR 72205, USA; [d] Silverado Senior Living, 330 North Hayworth Avenue, Los Angeles, CA 90048, USA; [e] Azusa Pacific University, School of Nursing, 701 East Foothill Boulevard, Building 1, Azusa, CA 91702-7000, USA
* Corresponding author.
E-mail address: dwoods@apu.edu

Nurs Clin N Am 57 (2022) 273–286
https://doi.org/10.1016/j.cnur.2022.02.009
0029-6465/22/© 2022 Elsevier Inc. All rights reserved.

severity of dementia is associated with increased negative consequences of social isolation, leading to a decrement in cognitive status and increased behavioral symptoms of dementia (BSD).[1] The aim of this paper is to examine the role of nursing leadership to address social isolation in LTC settings through evidence-based practices that protect and enhance the quality of life for residents with dementia. In addition, the paper will explore strategies to prevent social isolation, the importance of spiritual and cultural considerations, and the significance of interdisciplinary collaboration.

It must be noted that the lack of professional nursing leadership in LTC has been and remains a longstanding issue.[2,3] As noted by Harvath and colleagues,[4] most directors of nursing in LTC have graduated from a diploma or associate degree program with no leadership or specific gerontological training, rendering them ill equipped for these positions. Moreover, the bulk of care for some of these most complex older adults is provided by paraprofessionals with little targeted education to care for this vulnerable population. Indeed, poor management practices are associated with high staff turnover, creating major barriers to person-centered dementia care.[5] Lessons highlighted by the coronavirus pandemic include the realization that augmenting person-centered care is essential, as is interdisciplinary collaboration, such that comprehensive holistic care is not compromised. Best practices indicate mandatory activities and socialization, a need to continue these even in difficult circumstances.[6]

The Importance of Social Connectedness

Social connection is key for older adults' well-being. Family and friends are critical. Being socially engaged and connected influences psychological and emotional well-being as well as having a positive effect on physical health[7] and longevity.[8] Moreover, a lack of social engagement and connectedness is associated with negative health outcomes such as depression. In addition, actual and perceived social isolation is associated with an increased risk of mortality.[9] Furthermore, research over the past 15 years has indicated that social isolation is strongly associated with comorbid conditions such as hypertension, cardiovascular disease,[10,11] cognitive decline,[12] depression,[13] and early mortality.[14] Because of the impact of isolation on mental health and well-being, the World Health Organization cautioned about the use of the incorrect term "social distancing" that referred to increasing physical space between people. Instead they highlighted the need to refer to these measures as "physical distancing" and to conceptualize policies to avoid disconnection from family and loved ones because there is a pressing need to stay emotionally and socially connected.[15] Although this terminology is important to consider at any point in time, this became crucial during the COVID-19 pandemic. The extent to which an individual is socially connected depends on multiple factors, including structural, functional, and quality components.[16] Not only does one need to have social connections, the perceptions of these relationships are inextricably linked to the risk of developing loneliness and/or social isolation.

The 2020 Report of the Lancet Commission noted brain mechanisms responsible for enhancing or maintaining cognitive reserve and preventing dementia. One of the main factors is maintenance of frequent social contact.[17] Growing evidence indicates that the magnitude of the effect of social isolation on mortality risk is comparable to, or greater than, factors such as smoking, obesity, and physical inactivity.[16] In addition, social isolation not only increases the risk for dementia but is also associated with increased memory decline and increased behavioral symptoms in those with dementia.[18,19] Social isolation coupled with the sensory impairments associated with aging leads to a synergistic effect of more severe isolation. Social vulnerability, frailty, and mortality are a dangerous triad for older adults, especially those with dementia.[20]

An animal study completed by Muntsant and Giménez-Llort[21] highlighted brain changes in rodents that mimic brain changes in those with dementia as a result of social isolation. The study examined the impact of long-term social isolation on male 3xTg-AD mice modeling advanced stages of Alzheimer disease (AD) compared with age-matched counterparts with normal aging. The main findings were an exacerbated (2-fold increase) hyperactivity and emergence of bizarre behaviors in isolated 3xTg-AD mice, worrisome results, as agitation is a challenge in the clinical management of dementia and an important cause of caregiver burden. Asymmetric atrophy of the hippocampus (the area of the brain most associated with memory), recently described in human beings with dementia, was also found to increase with isolation. These results emphasize the negative consequences of isolation, consequences that are not only psychological but also profoundly physiologic. Moreover, they also highlight the relevance of personalized-based interventions tailored to the heterogeneous and complex clinical profile of the individuals with dementia and to consider the implications on caregiver burden.

THE CALL FOR NURSING LEADERSHIP
Where Do We Go from Here?

A post–COVID-19 era implies strong efforts to redesign living conditions and lifestyles, to find new care models, and to provide better management of the social isolation of residents enforced by physical distance; this requires leadership. Much of this isolation could have been prevented with educated and informed nursing leadership such that pandemic regulations could have been implemented while maintaining social engagement and connection.

Shared governance models provide structures and processes that empower frontline engagement in practice and policy decision-making.[22,23] The effectiveness of shared governance largely depends on supportive nursing leadership, providing an infrastructure that supports and empowers all staff to participate in clinical decision-making and work collaboratively to affect resident outcomes.[24] This participation is especially important for those who have been overlooked in LTC, the direct care workers (DCW).

Kanter's theory of structural empowerment[25] underscores how organizational performance benefits from leaders sharing power with employees through structures and processes that bolster access to information, resources, support, and professional development and learning opportunities.[26] This level of understanding and application requires professional nursing leadership in LTC to implement these principles.

In their narrative review, Zonneveld and Minkman[27] explored appropriate leadership in LTC. Overall they found that, although context dependent, relationship-oriented behaviors, where leaders focus on relationship, were significantly associated with the implementation of person-centered care and psychosocial climate. In contrast, high staff turnover and absences were related to less effective nursing leadership, whereas close interpersonal relationships were positively related to leadership. Corazzini and colleagues[28] describe adaptive leadership requiring new and innovative solutions, which may also require a change in values or attitudes. In this context, technical challenges refer to issues easily defined and solved with the appropriate expertise or resources. Issues often include both technical and adaptive challenges, in which different leadership behaviors are needed. Professional nursing leadership, those who are registered nurses (RNs), with leadership training at a minimum, can coordinate comprehensive assessment, advocate for resources, and coordinate with the interdisciplinary team to ensure high-quality care. The need for interdisciplinary collaboration, such as nursing, social work, rehabilitation services, medicine, and chaplaincy cannot be overemphasized. All members of the team can assess and plan to meet resident needs culturally, functionally, spiritually, and socially to prevent impairment during isolation.[29] In fact, interdisciplinary collaboration is essential for program success.

SOCIAL ENGAGEMENT PRACTICES

Nursing leadership has proved critical to the implementation of programs that focus on social engagement and connectedness. Using a Delphi consensus approach, Kales and colleagues[30] identified 4 targeted nonpharmacological approaches for those with dementia and BSD: caregiver/staff training, adaptation of the environment, person-centered care, and tailored activities, as first-line approaches before any pharmacologic approaches. These targeted approaches highlight the importance and value of nondrug approaches. In addition, the consensus was that DICE (Describe, Investigate, Create, Evaluate) was the preferred nondrug approach followed by music therapy.[30]

Kolanowski and colleagues[2] have suggested that affect balance may be used to assess well-being in persons with dementia. The Bradburn Scale of Psychological Well Being (Affect Balance Scale), first developed by Bradburn and Noll,[31] compares the frequency of positive affect with negative affect over a period of time. However, absence of negative affect does not equate with well-being. The higher the ratio of positive affect, the greater the well-being. Kolanowski and colleagues[32] found that modifiable factors such as positive staff interaction, number of RN hours, number of certified nurse assistant hours, and higher resident function were significantly associated with higher positive resident affect balance. Earlier work by Tappen and Williams[33] found an association between positive staff communication and resident mood supporting Kolanowski and colleagues'[34] findings. In addition, modifiable factors including the built environment, such as light, noise, and seating, can be supportive or provide barriers to optimal independence, physical activity, and well-being. The findings of Kales and colleagues[30] and Kolanowski and colleagues[35] have major implications for LTC staff education, specifically the importance of staff communication training during caregiving interactions. Communication training is an essential component to ensure the well-being of residents with dementia.

Bethell and colleagues[36] reviewed observational and intervention studies on social connections in LTC, finding associations with various mental health impacts. Among 61 studies the reported mental health outcomes included "depression; responsive behaviors; mood, affect, emotions; anxiety; boredom; suicidal thoughts; psychiatric morbidity; and daily crying" (p. 231) acknowledging overlap among categories. Bethell and colleagues[36] identified 12 strategies, informed by 72 observational studies that may help residents, families, and staff build on and maintain social connection. Findings included managing pain; addressing sensory needs (vision, hearing); sleep at night (vs daytime); opportunities for creative expression; exercise; maintaining religious and cultural practices; garden (indoor or outdoor); visits with pets; use technology to communicate; laugh together; reminisce about events, people, places; and address communication impairments and communicate nonverbally.[36] Critical barriers to successful implementation are chronic understaffing[36] and staff turnover that can be as high as 85% within many facilities.[37,38]

In a recent study with direct care workers (DCW) in LTC, Woods and colleagues found that teaching staff strategies including a method of approach and therapeutic communication increased their confidence in interacting with those with dementia in a positive manner and decreased their self-reported stress levels (Woods, unpublished data 2021). Moreover, DCW urinary oxytocin, a hormone that measures social bonding and connectedness, increased when DCW administered the CALM (therapeutic communication and therapeutic touch) intervention to residents (Woods, unpublished data 2021). In a 3-group experimental study, this calming intervention, therapeutic touch, showed a significant decrease in agitation for those with BSD.[39]

An early qualitative study by Thorne and colleagues[40] asked older adults about what the term "wellness" meant to them. Interviews with 15 older adults residing in LTC found 3 themes: comfort and abilities, connectedness and competence, and sense of meaning. A sense of meaning was found to be the foundation that cements the other dimensions of health and well-being, assertions that support Travelbee's[41] discussion about the importance of meaning in human experience. Although resident's spiritual and existential needs are acknowledged, they are frequently left to clergy and not institutionalized into any programming. Taking measures to understand what gives a resident meaning is essential to their health and well-being. The spiritual needs of these patients need to be addressed with appropriate interventions put into action. Spirituality can be defined as the belief in a power greater than self, which may or may not involve membership in a specific religion.[42] Some of the spiritual needs of older LTC residents during the pandemic were the need or desire to attend church with their family members, to commune with those of the same faith, and to participate in the community activities associated with attendance at religious services such as singing and receiving communion.[43]

LTC communities attempt to engage residents in stimulating activities and encourage social connections to add to quality of life.[44] During the pandemic restrictions group activities and person-to-person contact were stopped. Better attempts at continuing modified enrichment activities may have prevented the increase in depression and cognitive decline.[45,46]

The staff in LTC facilities are entrusted with caring for the most vulnerable at-risk older adults, a challenging mandate. A systematic review conducted by Seitz and colleagues[47] found that of 74 studies reviewed, the median prevalence for resident dementia was 58%, whereas the median prevalence of behavioral symptoms among those with dementia was 78%. Moreover, the median prevalence of depressive symptoms was 29%. These data were collected years before COVID-19. The restrictions of the pandemic worsened many of these issues, as visits to LTC facilities were banned, group activities ceased, and residents had no face-to-face contact with their families nor interaction with other residents. Residents were socially isolated, lacking the social and environmental enrichment that are key factors to mitigate cognitive decline and increased behavioral symptoms. Redistribution and relocation of rooms also contributed to increased stress and behavioral problems; each new arrangement resulted in residents adjusting to a new environment.[30,48] Coping with stress and negative and sad emotions has a stronger impact on older adults due to their age-related decrement on immune function and the neuro-immune dysregulation associated with these psychosocial processes.[49]

CULTURAL PERSPECTIVES

Cultural associations as we age are linked to feelings of belonging and mental well-being.[43] As we age these associations become an important connection to community and encourage socialization through shared worship, celebrations, and common languages.[43,50] Statistics on nursing home residents in the United States finds that of those 65 years and older, 81% were non-Hispanic White, 12% were African American,

5% Hispanic, and 2% as Asian/Pacific Islander.[51] Racial and cultural stigmas combined with privacy concerns are barriers to socialization as well as obstructions for health care professional access.[43]

Acculturation is more difficult later in life, and adjusting to living in a residential facility may be difficult for many.[50] The loss of social networks or work peers is associated with a higher risk of depression and anxiety in those of advanced years.[52] Many LTC staff are from different ethnic origins than the residents for whom they care, presenting challenges of communication among ethnically diverse LTC residents.[53] In 2015, Kim and colleagues found that culturally congruent communication, including verbal and nonverbal styles, between DCW and residents was associated with a decrease in behavioral symptoms for those with dementia, potentially because culturally congruent communication evoked a sense of familiarity and comfort. Culturally sensitive perspectives are imperative in providing quality of care for a rapidly changing, ethnically diverse aging population, modeled and supported by professional nursing leadership.

Nursing leadership in LTC must be cognizant of the impact that social isolation has not only for residents, but staff as well; caring for those older adults with dementia and those with different cultural backgrounds can be stressful for the LTC facility staff on any given day. Some of the stress that both residents and staff experience is related to divergent staff-resident communication culture, resulting in increased BSD.[54] Adding social isolation to the equation amplifies staff stress interfering with their ability to adequately provide the needed care for those with dementia, particularly focused on maintaining social connection and social engagement. Communication issues and strategies and education that increase cultural congruency should be key staff educational foci. Some strategies that address barriers to these issues can be incorporated into educational programs, for example, culturally specific verbal and nonverbal ways of greeting older adults, introducing oneself before beginning care, and using simple and familiar words; this is especially important for DCW who provide the bulk of the care, belong to an ethnic group different from the resident, and have little formal education.

Implementing interventions to address and support staff's stress is vital for the mental health of the valuable caregivers who have had to step up and take on multiple roles in providing care to help prevent social isolation, especially with residents with dementia. Cummings and colleagues[55] found that a higher level of staff job satisfaction corresponded to more effective leadership. Residential facilities that demonstrate adaptability, community approaches to challenges, and productive engagement of residents have been associated with healthier lifestyles.[56,57]

The multitude of deficits that characterize dementia add to the challenges that LTC facilities face to prevent social isolation. During the pandemic, staff and resident routines were disrupted such that staff, mainly DCW, were less able to provide activities that focused on connectedness and engagement such as socially focused group activities and cognitive stimulation or meet physical and psychosocial needs. Research has found that more health-related education and knowledge leads to increased participation in care and better overall outcomes.[56] Education on the deleterious effects of social isolation and the positive affect of cultural congruency in those with dementia needs to be disseminated to the staff at all levels.[58,59] Nursing leadership is essential to develop and implement programs that include this focus.

STAFF EDUCATION: AN ESSENTIAL INGREDIENT

Increasing staff's competencies and supporting and promoting an interdisciplinary collaborative culture among all staff, (DCWs, nurses, therapists, social workers, and family practitioners at a minimum) are essential in supporting persons living with dementia. Moreover, it is critical to increase staff knowledge and understanding about persons with dementia and their support networks. Interdisciplinary collaboration is essential thus learning how to collaborate within an interdisciplinary team from a person-centered care perspective, for example, is important. Another example of this collaboration involves developing interdisciplinary team meetings to review residents' care plans, especially including staff participation in these teams, especially DCW who may need encouragement to participate.

Fostering an environment that perpetuates open communication between staff and leadership lays the foundation for a healthy work environment. Conversations regarding staff perceptions of their workloads and needed education related to the care of residents with dementia is a starting point. Staff's ability to communicate with those with cognitively impaired residents is fundamental; however, some LTC facilities may be deficient in providing the education to staff about how to effectively connect with residents. Fundamentally, staff gain an understanding that their skills in communication build relationships and healthy interactions among these residents with communication impairments.[60]

In addition to providing ongoing staff education regarding caring for residents with dementia, nursing leadership needs to focus on decreasing staff turnover and improving workflow. Providing opportunities to support consistent staff assignments that create routines and relationships tailored toward individual resident's needs promotes the positive opportunities to be able to have adequate time to engage with residents and prevent their social isolation.

Changing the LTC facility culture to promote strategies to prevent social isolation can take time and effort. Nursing leadership is in a position to model the behaviors that demonstrate approaches to preventing social isolation, as well as supporting staff activities that engage residents in their care.[60] Setting expectations for the staff to engage in strategies that prevent resident exclusion, actually promoting social inclusion, helps pave the way to success. Doing so builds the relationships between staff and residents beyond attention solely based on clinical care.[62]

Nurse leaders in LTC must model leadership behaviors. Interacting with residents is important. These interactions can be implemented with daily leadership rounds involving both the resident and staff. Problem behaviors possibly linked to social isolation can be noted during the rounds, and a timely action plan can be developed involving the resident and staff to address the issue (Lehman, 2021). Holding focus groups with staff to identify their perceptions of success in preventing social isolation is a strategy leadership can implement. Who better to describe what is actually occurring than the staff who are with the residents for long periods, especially those with dementia? Involving staff to be a part of the solution to prevent social isolation is vital for success.[62]

PROGRAM EXEMPLAR ON ENGAGING AND CONNECTING

One program that includes recommendations by Kales and colleagues (2019)[30] and Andresen[61] is Nexus, an evidence-based model for memory care, showing a positive impact on cognition through social engagement and connectedness. The word *nexus* is derived from the Latin *nectere*, meaning "to bind or tie." The term often represents the point where different occurrences or ideas come together or intersect, a connection or series of connections linking two or more things. The Nexus program, developed by Andresen,[62] is an evidence-based program focused on optimizing cognitive functioning. The program includes a variety of activities categorized under 5 pillars of brain health: (1) physical exercise programs (walking clubs, dancing classes, morning workouts); (2) cognitive exercises (creative writing club, group word games); (3) stress reduction (chair yoga classes, group-guided meditation); (4) purposeful social activities (service club, cooking classes, making floral arrangements for the community), and (5) support groups. Nexus constitutes a model for staff training that increases staff competencies in dementia care through an interdisciplinary and cross-sectional classroom.[61]

Andresen[62] presented data on this innovative program at the Alzheimer Disease International Conference. Findings from 423 residents who scored greater than or equal to 15 on the Folstein Mini Mental State Exam (MMSE)[63] were included in the original study of 5 Danish LTC communities. Activities of daily living (ADLs) were measured using the Alzheimer Disease Cooperative Study—Activities of Daily Living (ADCS-ADL) every 6 months between September 1, 2015 and September 1, 2017. Ninety-one residents completed both measures at 6 months, 68 completed at 12 months, and 18 completed at 18 months. Findings indicate that those with the highest MMSE at baseline maintain or increase their cognitive function and ADLs over a period of 2 years lending credence for the use of social engagement and connectedness to not only combat isolation but also optimize cognitive function in adults with mild or major cognitive impairment in LTC.

Recently, Andresen[61] reported that after 6 months of focused workshops using the 5 pillars, staff when interviewed from 3 Danish nursing homes described increased awareness and feelings of being more successful when interviewed. Moreover, Andresen[61] assessed the Nexus Program in one LTC over a period of 2 years, finding that there was a 60% improvement in cognition, for those with an MMSE score greater than or equal to 20 compared with those who did not participate in the program, which supported clinical observations.

Several LTC facilities in the United States have adapted this structured and individualized approach for those with mild-to-moderate dementia in memory care. The Nexus program, planned by the social work and recreational activity staff, works in conjunction with the philosophy of person-centered care promoting optimal function in these specific LTCs. The residents, all of which have some form of cognitive impairment, spend most of the day out of their rooms. The staff help the residents get dressed and ready for the day, guiding them to the common areas. Residents may participate in varied groups, organized and supervised by social work and recreational staff, depending on their interests and cognitive ability. If a resident is socially withdrawing, it is an indicator that they are having difficulty keeping up with the group they are in, and the staff will introduce the resident to try a different group. Residents that are not actively engaged in a planned activity can still sit in common areas with other residents, reading in the library or watching television in the lounge.

Cheston and colleagues[64] describe dementia as an "existential threat" emphasizing the importance of maintaining a sense of identity and purpose in people with dementia. For this program to be effective, it is important for the staff to help residents to maintain this sense of identity and minimize the loss of self-described by Cohen and Eisdorfer[65] by understanding the residents as individuals. By knowing their likes and dislikes, staff can encourage their participation accordingly. Staff solicit brief profiles from families. Knowing the resident's past interests or career can help the resident continue to feel that they have a purpose in society. Shadow boxes outside resident rooms display photos and keepsakes from the resident's life. These help staff to be familiar with the resident's life and also act as reminders for the residents themselves. The environment can contribute enormously to a sense of self and connectedness, reflecting a feeling of normalcy and belonging, rather than segregation from society. Nexus LTC facilities often have pets such as dogs, cats, fish, and birds. In addition, staff and visitors encourage staff and visitors to bring their children to the facility so that they can also engage the residents.

Acquiring nutrition is part of social activity. Volkert and colleagues[66] provided recommendations about meeting the nutritional needs of individuals with dementia. Nexus program residents eat in a large dining room set up such as a restaurant with silverware and table cloths. Several residents, typically 3 or 4, or just 2 when physical distancing, are seated at each table; this provides the residents with social cues that promote good intake and encouragement to eat.

Another important component of the model of care is music. Baird and Thompson[67] examined how music helps combat the disruption to one's sense of self that people with dementia often experience. Their work found that music has the capability to engage individuals in a uniquely holistic way. With such a highly stigmatized disease, music has a critical ability to affirm the identity of the individual rather than letting the person being defined simply by their diagnosis. These LTC communities have live musical entertainment on a regular basis. At one LTC, the Director of Resident Engagement is a board-certified music therapist, with music therapy interns working one-to-one with residents as well as playing for the group. The music therapist also leads the resident choir, who practice weekly and perform regularly for the community. Beyond the choir, the musicians routinely encourage the residents to sing along as they play music, which makes music a social activity where residents can enjoy each other's company people and learn they love the same songs.

Focus groups with residents asking what is going well encourages their involvement in strategies that promote social engagement and is another approach to preventing social isolation. Assessing the needs and desires of the LTC resident helps to personalize interactions and can lead to encouraging resident engagement in activities geared toward promoting social inclusion. For those residents with dementia or other cognitive impairments who may not be able to provide this information, asking family and friends can elicit important information specifically individualized for this resident. Gaining this information, in whatever forum, helps leadership develop and secure resources for the facility to enhance greater social engagement.

An LTC facility social worker from Southern California reported that 28 residents were participating in the NEXUS Program in January 2021. From those 28, 19 (68%) remained in the program after 6 months. Six residents (21%) were withdrawn from the program, as they no longer met the MMSE greater than or equal to 20, and the remainder (11%) left the program due to a move from the facility or death (M. Dawson, personal communication, July 9, 2021).

IMPLICATIONS MOVING FORWARD

Nursing leaders have a responsibility to promote and facilitate social engagement and connectedness to mitigate social isolation in LTC. The 2020 to 2021 COVID-19 pandemic emphasized longstanding problems in LTC facilities, such as staff mix, workload, and support. Moreover, the pandemic shed light on the severe deleterious effect of social isolation and the critical importance of maintaining social engagement and connectedness especially in times of crisis or major change. Staff education and ongoing support cannot be overemphasized. Critical nursing leadership and interdisciplinary collaboration engaging all team members is essential in operationalizing non-pharmacological approaches that foster the well-being of residents with dementia.

LTC settings are complex systems with nursing leadership, an essential component for improved resident outcomes, especially those most vulnerable residents with dementia. The presence of nurse leaders in LTC with more experience is associated with a decreased prevalence of BSD, improved mobility, greater relationship-oriented leadership practices, higher levels of open communication between DSW and management staff[68] and less staff turnover.[69] A National Hartford Center of Gerontological Nursing Excellence funded training program, consisting of both leadership and gerontological content was delivered to 14 nurse managers in the Veteran's Health Administration (VHA) Community Living Centers (CLC). Results showed an improvement in quality indicators such as function (78.6%) and decreased antipsychotic medications (76.9%) over a 6-month period (Kolanowski and colleagues,[34] personal communication, July 14, 2021). These results support the development and mandating of specific dedicated programs that address the deficits in nursing leadership and gerontological knowledge in LTC. Staff education and ongoing support cannot be overemphasized. For example, group meetings to talk about staff challenges and find resolutions specifically effective communication. Nursing leadership and interdisciplinary collaboration are critical, engaging all team members to develop coordinated programs to foster dementia well-being is critical.

The strategies delineated earlier that emphasize education, positive interactions and connectedness with residents, and bonding and well-being are associated with decreased staff stress, increased job satisfaction, and decreased staff turnover. Moreover, programs such as Nexus can be expanded to incorporate the national Age-Friendly Health System's initiative including the evidence-based 4 Ms (What Matters, Medication, Mentation, and Mobility)[70–73] with a focus on what matters, an essential component, as Travelbee[41] and Thorne and colleagues[40] noted several years ago. Now implementation of key nursing leadership strategies is essential to avoid further crises and promote social connectivity in LTC.

CLINICS CARE POINTS

- Incorporate social engagement programs especially for those with dementia to optimize cognitive and physical functioning.
- Establish resident group activities by level of cognitive impairment for optimal resident engagement.
- Educate staff about resident's life, accomplishments, and interests to facilitate connectedness.
- Use meals as a social activity to create opportunities for connection and improve nutritional intake.
- Incorporate music to engage residents in group and individual settings.
- Use shared cultural traditions such as worship, celebrations, and other common languages during times of mandated isolation to increase engagement and connectedness.
- Nursing leadership in LTC is essential to understand and communicate the impact that social isolation has not only for residents but staff as well.

DISCLOSURE

The authors have nothing to disclose.

REFERENCES

1. Dourado MCN, Belfort T, Monteiro A, de Lucena AT, Lacerda IB, Gaigher J, Baptista MAT, Brandt M, Kimura NR, de Souza N, Gasparini P, Rangel R, Marinho V.

COVID-19: challenges for dementia care and research. Dement Neuropsychol. 2020 Dec;14(4):340–44. https://doi.org/10.1590/1980-57642020dn14-040002. PMID: 33354285; PMCID: PMC7735054.

2. Kolanowski A, Cortes TA, Mueller C, et al. A call to the CMS: Mandate adequate professional nurse staffing in nursing homes. Am J Nurs 2021;121(3):24–7.
3. Levac D, Colquhoun H, O'Brien KK. Scoping studies: advancing the methodology. Implementations Sci 2010;5(1):69.
4. Harvath TA, Swafford K, Smith K, et al. Enhancing nursing leadership in long-term care: A review of the literature. Res Gerontological Nurs 2008;1(3):187–96.
5. Resnick B, Galik E, Vigne E, Carew AP. Dissemination and Implementation of Function Focused Care for Assisted Living. Health Educ Behav. 2016 Jun;43(3):296-304. https://doi.org/10.1177/1090198115599984. Epub 2015 Aug 26. PMID: 27178495.
6. Hwang T-J, Rabheru K, Peisah C, et al. Loneliness and social isolation during the COVID-19 pandemic. Int Psychogeriatrics 2020;32(10):1217–20.
7. Uchino BN. Social support and health: a review of physiological processes potentially underlying links to disease outcomes. J Behav Med 2006 Aug;29(4): 377–87. https://doi.org/10.1007/s10865-006-9056-5.
8. Holt-Lunstad J, Smith TB, Layton JB. Social relationships and mortality risk: a meta-analytic review. PLoS Med 2010 Jul 27;7(7). https://doi.org/10.1371/journal.pmed.1000316. PMID: 20668659; PMCID: PMC2910600.
9. Holt-Lunstad J, Smith TB, Baker M, Harris T, Stephenson D. Loneliness and social isolation as risk factors for mortality: a meta-analytic review. Perspect Psychol Sci. 2015 Mar;10(2):227–37. https://doi.org/10.1177/1745691614568352. PMID: 25910392.
10. Arthur HM. Depression, isolation, social support, and cardiovascular disease in older adults. J Cardiovasc Nurs 2006;21(5/1):S2–7.
11. Cacioppo JT, Hawkley LC. Social isolation and health, with an emphasis on underlying mechanisms. Perspect Biol Med 2003;45(3):S39–52.
12. Read S, Comas-Herrera A, Grundy E. Social isolation and memory decline in later- life. J Gerontol B Psychol Sci Soc Sci 2020;75(2):367–76.
13. Paul C, Ayis S, Ebrahim S. Psychological distress, loneliness and disability in old age. Psychol Health Med 2006;11(2):221–32.
14. Gerst Emerson K, Jayawardhana J. Loneliness as a public health issue: The impact of loneliness on health care utilization among older adults. Am J Public Health 2015;105:1013–9.
15. World Health Organization. COVID-19: physical distancing. Available at: https://www.who.int/westernpacific/emergencies/covid-19/information/physical-distancing. Accessed May 23, 2021.
16. National Academies of Sciences, Engineering, and medicine. Social isolation and loneliness in older adults: opportunities for the health care system. Washington, D. C.: The National Academies Press; 2020.
17. Livingston G, Huntley J, Sommerlad A, et al. Dementia prevention, intervention, and care: 2020 report of the Lancet Commission. Lancet 2020;396(10248): 413–46.
18. Friedler B, Crapser J, McCullough L. One is the deadliest number: the detrimental effects of social isolation on cerebrovascular diseases and cognition. Acta Neuropathol 2015;129:493–509.
19. Wilson RS, Krueger KR, Arnold SE, et al. Loneliness and risk of Alzheimer disease. Arch Gen Psychiatry 2007;64(2):234–40.

20. Andrew MK, Mitnitski AB, Rockwood K. Social vulnerability, frailty, and mortality in elderly people. PLoS One 2008;3(5):e2232.

21. Muntsant A, Giménez-Llort L. Impact of social isolation on the behavioral, functional profiles, and hippocampal atrophy asymmetry in dementia in times of coronavirus pandemic (COVID-19): A translational neuroscience approach. Front Psychiatry 2020;11. Article 572583. https://doi/10.3389/fpsyt.2020.572583.

22. Anthony MK. Shared governance models: The theory, practice, and evidence. Online J Issues Nurs 2004;9(1):7.

23. Arksey H, O'Malley L. Scoping studies: Towards a methodological framework. Int J Social Res Methodol 2005;8(1):19–32.

24. Hess R. Shared governance is everywhere! Insight. J Am Soc Ophthalmic Registered Nurses 2020;45(3):37–9.

25. Kanter R. Men and women of the corporation. New York: Basic Books; 1977.

26. Clavelle JT, O'Grady TP, Weston M, et al. Evolution of structural empowerment: Moving from shared to professional governance. J Nurs Adm 2016;46(6):308–12.

27. Zonneveld N, Pittens C, Minkman M. Appropriate leadership in nursing home care: a narrative review. Leadersh Health Serv (Bradf Engl). 2021 Mar 22;ahead-of-print(ahead-of-print):16–36. https://doi.org/10.1108/LHS-04-2020-0012. PMID: 33738993; PMCID: PMC8317028.

28. Corazzini K, Twersky J, White HK, et al. Implementing culture change in nursing homes: An adaptive leadership framework. Gerontologist 2015;55(4):616–27.

29. Parekh de Campos A, Daniels S. Ethical implications of COVID-19: Palliative care, public health, and long-term care facilities. J Hosp Palliat Nurs 2021;23(2):120–7.

30. Kales HC, Lyketsos CG, Miller EM, et al. Management of behavioral and psychological symptoms in people with Alzheimer's disease: an international delphi consensus. Int Psychogeriatr 2019;31:83–90.

31. Bradburn NM, Noll CE. The structure of psychological well-being. Chicago: Aldine; 1969.

32. Kolanowski A, Behrens L, Lehman E, et al. Living well with dementia: Factors associated with nursing home residents' affect balance. Res Gerontological Nurs 2020;13(1):21–30.

33. Tappen RM, Williams CL. Therapeutic conversation to improve mood in nursing home residents with Alzheimer's disease. Res Gerontol Nurs. 2009 Oct;2(4):267–75. https://doi.org/10.3928/19404921-20090428-02. Epub 2009 Oct 27. PMID: 20077983.

34. Kolanowski AM, Van Haitsma K, Meeks S, et al. Affect balance and relationship with well-being in nursing home residents with dementia. Am J Alzheimer's Other Demen 2014;29(5):457–62.

35. Kolanowski A, Cortes TA, Mueller C, Bowers B, Boltz M, Bakerjian D, Harrington C, Popejoy L, Vogelsmeier A, Wallhagen M, Fick D, Batchelor M, Harris M, Palan Lopez R, Dellefield M, Mayo A, Woods DL, Horgas A, Cacchione PZ, Carter D, Tabloski P, Gerdner L. A call to the CMS: Mandate adequate professional nurse staffing in nursing homes. American Journal of Nursing 2021;121(3):24–7. https://doi.org/10.1097/01.NAJ.0000737292.96068.18. PMID: 33625007.

36. Bethell J, Aelick K, Babineau J, et al. Social connection in long- term care homes: A scoping review of published research on the mental health impacts and potential strategies during COVID-19. J Am Med Dir Assoc 2021;22:228–37.

37. Castle NG, Engberg J. Staff turnover and quality of care in nursing homes. Med Care 2005;43(6):616–26.

38. Donoghue C, Castle N. Organizational and environmental effects on voluntary and involuntary turnover. Health Care Manage Rev 2007;32(4):360–9.
39. Woods DL, Craven R, Whitney J. The effect of therapeutic touch on behavioral symptoms of persons with dementia. Altern Ther Health Med 2005;11(1):66–74.
40. Thorne S, Griffin C, Adlersberg M. Well seniors' perceptions of their health and well-being. How's your health? Gerontion 1986;1(5):15–8.
41. Travelbee J. To find meaning in illness. Nursing 1972;2(12):6–8.
42. Toivonen K, Charalambous A, Suhonen R. Supporting spirituality in the care of older people living with dementia: a hermeneutic phenomenological inquiry into nurses' experiences. Scand J Caring Sci 2018;32(2):880–8.
43. Giwa S, Mullings DV, Karki KK. Virtual social work care with older Black adults: A culturally relevant technology-based intervention to reduce social isolation and loneliness in a time of pandemic. J Gerontol Soc Work 2020;63(6/7):679–81.
44. Oliver EJ, Hudson J, Thomas L. Processes of identity development and behaviour change in later life: Exploring self-talk during physical activity uptake. Ageing & Society 2016;36(7):1388–406. https://doi.org/10.1017/S0144686X15000410.
45. Nielsen K, Christensen M. Positive Participatory Organizational Interventions: A Multilevel Approach for Creating Healthy Workplaces. Front Psychol. 2021 Jun 28;12:696245. https://doi.org/10.3389/fpsyg.2021.696245. PMID: 34262513; PMCID: PMC8273334.
46. Temkin-Greener H, Guo W, Mao Y, Cai X, Li Y. COVID-19 Pandemic in Assisted Living Communities: Results from Seven States. Journal of the American Geriatrics Society 2020;68(12):2727–34. https://doi.org/10.1111/jgs.16850.
47. Seitz D, Purandare N, Conn D. Prevalence of psychiatric disorders among older adults in long-term care homes: A systematic review. Int Psychogeriatrics 2010;22(7):1025–39.
48. Wang H, Li T, Barbarino P, et al. Dementia care during COVID-19. Lancet 2020;395:1190–1.
49. Kiecolt-Glaser JK, McGuire L, Robles TF, et al. Psychoneuroimmunology and psychosomatic medicine: Back to the future. Psychosomatic Med 2002;64:15–28.
50. Chao YY, Li M, Lu SE, Dong X. Elder mistreatment and psychological distress among U.S. Chinese older adults. J Elder Abuse Negl. 2020 Nov-Dec;32(5):434–52. https://doi.org/10.1080/08946566.2020.1814180. Epub 2020 Sep 4. PMID: 32886054; PMCID: PMC7736261.
51. Li Y, Cai X, Harrington C, et al. Racial and ethnic differences in the prevalence of depressive symptoms among U.S. nursing home residents. J Aging Soc Policy 2019;31(1):30–48.
52. Zhang C, Zhao H, Zhu R, Lu J, Hou L, Yang XY, Yin M, Yang T. Improvement of social support in empty-nest elderly: results from an intervention study based on the Self-Mutual-Group model. Journal of public health (Oxford, England) 2019;41(4):830–9. https://doi.org/10.1093/pubmed/fdy185.
53. Kim H, Woods DL, Mentes JC, et al. The nursing assistants' communication style and the behavioral symptoms of dementia in Korean-American nursing home residents. Geriatr Nurs 2014;35(2):S11–6.
54. Kim H, Woods DL, Phillips LR, et al. Nursing assistants' communication styles in Korean American older adults with dementia: A review of the literature. J Transcult Nurs 2015;26(2):185–92.
55. Cummings G, Mallidou AA, Masaoud E, et al. On becoming a coach: a pilot intervention study with managers in long-term care. Health Care Manage Rev 2014;39(3):198–209.

56. Chantakeeree C, Sormunen M, Jullamate P, et al. Health-promoting behaviors among urban and rural older Thai adults with hypertension: a cross-sectional study. Pac Rim Int J Nurs Res 2021;25(2):242–54.
57. Gardiner C, Geldenhuys G, Gott M. Interventions to reduce social isolation and loneliness among older people: an integrative review. Health Soc Care Community 2018;26(2):147–57.
58. Ehrlich H, McKenney M, Elkbuli A. The need for actions to protect our geriatrics and maintain proper care at U.S. long-term care facilities. J Trauma Nurs 2020; 27(4):193–4.
59. Fakoya OA, McCorry NK, Donnelly M. Loneliness and social isolation interventions for older adults: A scoping review of reviews. BMC Public Health 2020; 20(1):129.
60. Leaman MC, Azios JH. Experiences of Social Distancing During Coronavirus Disease 2019 as a Catalyst for Changing Long-Term Care Culture. Am J Speech Lang Pathol. 2021 Jan 27;30(1):318–23. https://doi.org/10.1044/2020_AJSLP-20-00176. Epub 2021 Jan 5. PMID: 33400556.
61. Andresen M, Tremmel G, Lolland K, et al. Small changes made big differences: the organization, form, content and results of a 6- month pilot in three Danish nursing homes. Reykjavik (Iceland): Nordic Congress of Gerontology; 2021.
62. Andresen M. (2018, July 26) Nexus – Impact on cognition and ADL in long term memory care of an evidence-based model for memory care. 33rd International Conference of Alzheimer's Disease International, Chicago, USA.
63. Folstein MF, Folstein SE, McHugh PR. Mini-mental state". A practical method for grading the cognitive state of patients for the clinician. J Psychiatr Res 1975; 12(3):189–98.
64. Cheston R, Christopher G, Ismail S. Dementia as an existential threat: The importance of self-esteem, social connectedness and meaning in life. Sci Prog 2015; 98(4):416–9.
65. Cohen D, Eisdorfer C. The loss of self: a family resource for the care of Alzheimer's and related disorders. New York: W. W. Norton & Company; 2002.
66. Volkert D, Chourdakis M, Faxen-Irving G, et al. ESPEN guidelines on nutrition in dementia. Clin Nutr 2015;34(6):1052–73.
67. Baird A, Thompson WF. The impact of music on the self in dementia. J Alzheimer's Dis 2018;61(3):827–41.
68. Anderson RA, Issel LM, McDaniel RR Jr. Nursing homes as complex adaptive systems: Relationship between management practices and resident outcomes. Nurs Res 2013;52(1):12–21.
69. Donoghue C, Castle NG. Leadership styles of nursing home administrators and their association with staff turnover. Gerontologist. 2009 Apr;49(2):166–74. https://doi.org/10.1093/geront/gnp021. Epub 2009 Mar 27. PMID: 19363012.
70. Institute for Healthcare Improvement. Age-friendly health systems. Available at: http://www.ihi.org/Engage/Initiatives/Age-Friendly-Health-Systems/Pages/default.aspx. Accessed May 23, 2021.
71. Kales HC, Gitlin LN, Lyketsos CG. Management of neuropsychiatric symptoms of dementia in clinical settings: recommendations from a multidisciplinary expert panel. J Am Geriatr Soc 2014;62(4):762–9.
72. Kales HC, Gitlin LN, Lyketsos CG. State of the art review: Assessment and management of behavioral and psychological symptoms of dementia. Br Med J 2015; 350. https://doi.org/10.1136/bmj.h369. Article h369.
73. Mate K, Fulmer T, Pelton L, et al. Evidence for the 4Ms: Interactions and outcomes across the health care continuum. J Aging Health 2021;33(7):469–81.

Leading Improvements in the Delivery of Nursing Care for Older Adults with Frailty in Long-Term Care Using Mitchell's Quality Health Outcome Model and Health Outcome Data

Deanna Gray-Miceli, PhD, GNP-BC, FGSA, FAAN[a],*,
Pamela B. de Cordova, PhD, RN-BC[b], Jeannette A. Rogowski, PhD[c],
Laurie Grealish, RN, PhD, FACN[d]

KEYWORDS

- Frailty • Geriatric syndromes • Quality metrics • Nursing leadership • Nursology
- Failure to maintain

KEY POINTS

- Clinical characteristics of frailty and geriatric syndromes among residents are tabulated monthly to establish a benchmark for improvement by nurse leaders.
- Use of quality metrics indicators by nurse leaders inform the delivery of quality nursing care.
- Use of nurse competencies help direct patient centered interventions to improve the delivery of nursing care, resulting in resident safety and quality care.

INTRODUCTION

The long-term care (LTC) industry provides several types of services to assist older adults to achieve optimal levels of health, function, and overall well-being. LTC services encompass short-term rehabilitation, subacute level, assisted living,

[a] Thomas Jefferson University, Jefferson College of Nursing, 901 Walnut Street #707, Philadelphia, PA 19107, USA; [b] Rutgers, The State University of New Jersey, School of Nursing, Ackerson Hall, 180 University Avenue, Room 244, Newark, NJ 07102, USA; [c] The Pennsylvania State University, University Park, Pennsylvania, PA 16802, USA; [d] Subacute and Aged Nursing, Nursing & Midwifery, Menzies Health Institute Queensland, Griffith University and Nursing & Midwifery Education and Research Unit, Gold Coast Hospital & Health Services, Griffith University, Southport, Queensland 4215, Australia
* Corresponding author.
E-mail address: Deanna.Gray-Miceli@jefferson.edu

Nurs Clin N Am 57 (2022) 287–297
https://doi.org/10.1016/j.cnur.2022.02.007   nursing.theclinics.com
0029-6465/22/© 2022 Elsevier Inc. All rights reserved.

and LTC. These services commonly, but not always, provide professional nursing care 24 hours per day, with the exception of, depending on the state, assisted living. Across the United States, nearly 1.3 million persons more than the age of 65 years enter into LTC for assistance in the management of their health conditions[1] reliant on the care provided by interprofessional teams led by registered nurses (RNs).

As many of the recipients of nursing care in LTC facilities are older Medicare or Medicaid beneficiaries, the Centers for Medicare and Medicaid (CMS) monitors the provision of quality care metrics to its members. The CMS's Quality Metric database[2] provides one set of nurse-sensitive indicators of quality care recognized by public health authorities (Agency for Healthcare Research and Quality [AHRQ,[3]] as critical to the delivery of quality care and resident safety.

Besides CMS, the delivery of quality nursing care is regulated by state licensing agencies, as well as individually by professional nurses who follow practice standards of care according to their scope of practice and licensure.[4] Professional nurses deliver care, guided by the nursing meta-paradigm, with focused attention to human beings, environment, health, and nursing goals.[5] Attention to this broad meta-paradigm by professional nurses helps to ensure that health deficiencies within these respected domains are minimized. Adherence to nursing standards of practice, regulations, and the nursing meta-paradigm, creates an ideal environment to deliver the best possible outcomes for older consumers, the recipient of the delivery of nursing care. However, as our society continues to age, the demography of the LTC population and environment is changing, with more frail older adults with multiple medical problems. Multi-morbidity includes advanced complex illness, acute exacerbations of conditions, new onset of geriatric syndromes, and frailty. In light of the changing demographics of LTC service users, there is an opportunity for nursing leaders to champion the delivery of quality nursing care to this most vulnerable, and often frail, population.

Frailty is related to multimorbidity,[6] and those with frailty may also experience socioeconomic deprivation and increased mortality,[7] as well as decreased quality of life and health-related quality of life in LTC .[8,9] Therefore, it is imperative that frailty be identified and appropriately managed by nurse leaders working in LTC. Of particular importance for the attention of nurse leaders, is the identification of practice gaps that may contribute to complications or geriatric syndromes in people who are experiencing frailty.

The aim of this article is to describe how nurse leaders can use a conceptual framework to guide the identification of practice gaps and associated key leadership competencies to enact practice change for improved quality of care for people experiencing frailty. We provide an overview of the conceptual framework guiding how the person and the situation are viewed, which informs the nursing care provided, how nurse-sensitive outcome measures from the CMS Quality Metrics database can be used to identify potential gaps in nursing care, show how the model can be adapted to monitor frailty, and provide a CASE study to illustrate how key leadership competencies can be exercised to improve service delivery quality for LTC residents experiencing frailty. Practice gaps can be attributed to individual practice, but more often can be attributed to complexities in organizational systems and processes. Therefore, understanding the context influencing the delivery of nursing care in health care organizations is essential. Delivery of fundamental quality care to physically fragile older residents and those with complex care needs is achievable when nurse leaders are focused on identifying the dynamic factors operant within a health care organization that influence nursing care delivery.

CONCEPTUAL FRAMEWORK AND PRACTICE DELIVERY MODELS OF CARE

Mitchell's Quality Health Outcomes Model is a dynamic, multidimensional framework of contextual factors operative within health care systems that impact the delivery of care. It has been modified for LTC settings (refer to **Fig. 1**;[10]). This framework illustrates the structures, resources, and policy domains influencing the delivery of nursing care to vulnerable populations which expose potential practice gaps within the LTC facility, and that create opportunities for improvement in nursing care delivery.

The health outcomes within Mitchell's Quality Health Outcomes Model are noted to be interdependent on the surrounding multidimensional contextual factors that include:

1. The demographic and health characteristics of older NH residents;
2. System characteristics within the LTC facility influencing the delivery of professional nursing care, such as nurse practice environment, skill mix, and staffing ratios;
3. Process of care characteristics influencing the delivery of nursing care goals and intervention; and
4. Adverse outcomes including readmission rates and resident quality of life.

These 4 contextual factors broadly represent the nursing meta-paradigm of the human being, environment, nursing goals, and health.[5] Demographic and health characteristics of the human being embody "person," system characteristics and external

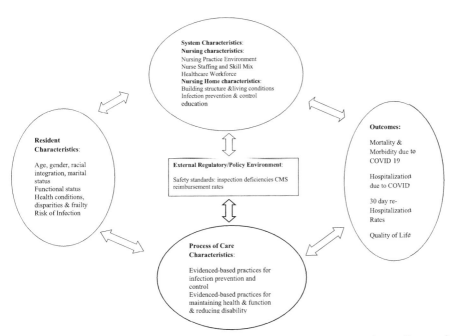

Fig. 1. Conceptual Relationship Among Contextual Factors Impacting the Delivery of Nursing Care in Nursing Homes Based on the Quality Health Outcomes Model (Mitchell, 1998). (*From* Gray-Miceli D, Rogowski J, de Cordova PB, Boltz M. A framework for delivering nursing care to older adults with COVID-19 in nursing homes. Public Health Nurs. 2021;00:1–17. https://doi.org/10.1111/phn.12885; with permission.)

regulatory characteristics embody "environment," process of nursing care embody "nursing goals" and adverse health outcomes embody "health."

Nursing assessment of these 4 contextual factors is an important role of the professional nurse leader within the health care organization. This conceptual framework reflects how the person and the situation are viewed, which then direct what nurse leaders and nursologists think about, and does with, for each person.[11,12] Nursologists use theory such as Roy's Adaptation Model or Neuman's Systems Model to frame how the person and their situation are viewed. The way by which nursing is delivered to persons occurs through various practice delivery models such as primary nursing, team nursing, or patient-centered care, among others.[11] Through nursing assessment, gaps in the delivery of nursing care can be identified and nursing care goals established to embrace the person, environment, and nursing goals for improved health outcomes. Nurse leaders in LTC facilities can develop effective nursing care interventions to manage the clinical nuances associated with frailty and burgeoning geriatric syndromes. Therefore, this review providers nurse leaders with the existing evidence from the QM database to illustrate how one symptom of frailty, coupled with structure, or process of care resources impacts health outcomes.

USING CENTERS FOR MEDICARE AND MEDICAID QUALITY METRICS TO IDENTIFY POTENTIAL GAPS IN NURSING CARE

To illustrate how to maximize leadership opportunities for nurses charged with the resident's care, we present nurse-sensitive Quality Metric[2] indicators among an older resident with symptoms of frailty along with 3 broad contextual factors that have impacted the delivery of quality care to this resident (ie, organizational and systems-level factors, resident characteristics and nursing interventions-process of care factors).

The Importance of Looking for Practice Gaps

A gap in care exists when the desired performance levels (ie, goals of care), are unaligned with current performance (ie, actual nursing care).[13] Gaps in care can lead to reduced remuneration to the LTC facility, loss of time to the resident to achieve their goals, health complications and geriatric syndromes that can lead to fines levied by state licensing inspection agencies and more importantly, inadequate quality resident outcomes. For example, researchers have identified the relationship between specific gaps in nursing care and adverse outcomes including pneumonia, urinary tract infection, pressure injury and delirium have been grouped together in the concept of "failure to maintain."[14] Not undertaking fundamental nursing care contributes to the development of these hospital-acquired complications, which are sometimes identified as geriatric syndromes.

Frailty and Cascade Iatrogenesis

Frailty is defined as "a state of vulnerability to poor resolution of homoeostasis after a stressor event, as a consequence of cumulative decline in many physiologic systems during a lifetime."[15] Frailty impacts the physical functional ability of an older resident. Considering their symptom experiences of exhaustion, low physical activity, and slowed speed of gait predisposes the older resident to need additional time to perform an activity as well as additional assistance to perform the activity safely. When it comes to the fundamental activities of daily living such as, transferring, ambulation, bathing, dressing, toileting, and feeding, more than 90% of residents have greater disability requiring assistance compared with noninstitutionalized older adults (US Census Bureau, 2017). Physical frailty is also associated with activities of daily living such as the ability to move independently, and thus it is important to recognize various degrees or severities progressing along a continuum of functional limitation and decline, from needing active assistance to move, to complete dependency-unable to move to perform the activity. Older residents who are bedridden may no longer possess the muscular strength or energy to move independently in bed, increasing their need for help with daily activities.

When homoeostatic reserves are depleted, and minor stressor events occur, they trigger disproportionate changes in older adult's health.[15] The older resident population in LTC facilities experience acute episodic changes in condition, considered "stressor events," that are often not specific to their underlying disease,[16] in addition to the burden of their chronic multi-morbidities. Weight loss, exhaustion, reduced grip strength, low physical activity, and slow walking pace are the 5 hallmark characteristics of frailty.[15] Two of the 5 symptoms, exhaustion and reduced physical activity, are also associated with the development of a preventable type of fall, which is recognized as a geriatric syndrome. Both exhaustion and reduced physical activity, left untreated, give rise to muscular weakness, loss of muscle mass that is, sarcopenia, and further reduced mobility and immobility, 2 additional preventable geriatric syndromes. Should fall episodes continue without improvement in resident's symptoms of exhaustion or physical activity, inevitable changes in upright mobility occur leading to further reduced mobility and immobility? Bedridden older residents are then at high risk for the development of pressure injury and/or nosocomial infection of the pressure injury. An event in one body system "can trigger larger complications or outcomes in another, or cascade iatrogenesis, among older adults with complex, high acuity needs."[17] Monitoring physical frailty and adverse outcomes related to the development of geriatric syndromes can be accomplished through the identification of nurse-sensitive quality metric data.

Monitoring Practice Gaps in Relation to Frailty

The CMS Quality Metric database (NH compare data. Medicare.gov) provides a range of metrics that could be considered sensitive to nursing care. These quality metrics are tabulated quarterly within all LTC facilities, across the states, serving as a gauge to monitor their quality improvement performance efforts to achieve resident safety and quality of care. To monitor the prevalence of frailty in a facility, the key primary outcome indicators captured in the CMS Quality Metric database most theoretically aligned to functional decline and/or worsening physical frailty include LTC residents' ability to move independently and an increase in needing help in activities of daily living (refer to **Box 1**).

CASE STUDY OF NURSING LEADERSHIP IN QUALITY IMPROVEMENT

The resident, Mrs G. (pseudonym), is an 86-year-old woman, recently widowed, who is admitted to the LTC facility, in an assisted living unit, for the management of her medications and assistance with activities of daily living. The characteristics of this CASE are outlined using the 4 meta-paradigm concepts: person, environment, nursing care, and health and illustrated in **Fig. 2**.

Person: Mrs G

Mrs G's medical history includes comorbidities of advanced coronary artery disease, peripheral vascular disease, multi-infarct dementia, and high-risk status for the

Box 1	
Example of some Quality Metrics linked to frailty in long-stay residents	
Quality Metric Number	**Quality Metric Definition**
QM 401	The percentage of long-stay residents whose need for help with daily activities has increased
QM 404	The percentage of long-stay residents who lose too much weight
QM 410	The percentage of long-stay residents experiencing one or more falls with major injury
QM 451	The percentage of residents whose ability to move independently worsened.
QM 453	The percentage of long-stay residents with pressure ulcers (injury)
QM 521	The number of outpatient emergency department visits per 1000 long-stay resident days

development of infection, related to an underlying immunodeficiency. Her current symptoms experienced include physical exhaustion after ambulation in her room for more than 15 feet with assistance, and decreased participation on the unit in physical activities such as group exercises, stretching, and chair yoga. She does not participate regularly in group exercises because she forgets. Mrs G's physical functional ability reveals dependency in mobility-using a wheeled walker for assistance, grooming, dressing, and toileting-experiencing stress urinary incontinence. She is able to select her clothes and feed herself. Her short-term rehabilitation goals are to: ambulate without the use of the wheeled walker:increase her lower extremity strength, and; stay at the facility for her remaining years.

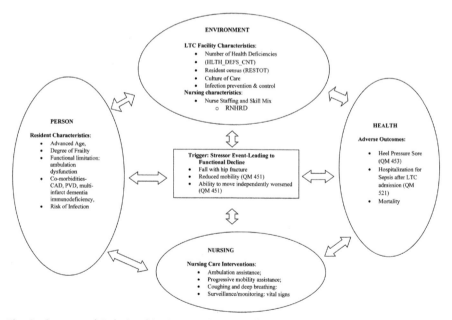

Fig. 2. Conceptual Relationship Among Contextual Factors Impacting the Continuum of Functional Decline Based on the Quality Health Outcomes Model (Mitchell, 1998). (*Data from* Dr. Gray-Miceli, copyright, 2021, all rights reserved.)

Trigger event and stressor event leading to functional decline. While ambulating with the physical therapy aide on the unit, Mrs G experiences a fall and is subsequently diagnosed with an acute fragility fracture in her right hip. Following surgery at the local hospital, she attends rehabilitation for 6 weeks at a short-term stay rehabilitation unit, to regain her strength and physical mobility before returning to the LTC unit. On readmission to the skilled nursing unit, Mrs G is physically exhausted by activities such as sitting on the side of bed or transferring from her bed to bedside chair for meals. Her ability to turn herself independently in bed is drastically reduced and she requires the assistance from the nursing staff to turn and position her.

Environment: Organizational Level Characteristics

The 110-bed skilled nursing unit whereby Mrs G resides has received on average four health deficiencies related to failure to administer meals and prescription medications during 2020. The facility is a privately owned chain facility, with 60% of the residents receiving Medicaid, and the remaining residents being dual-eligible for Medicare and Medicaid. The average resident census is full capacity at 110 beds. The CASE mix staffing hours per resident day is 0.36 as noted on the Quality Metric CM-RN. This is a measure of staffing and reimbursement for nursing based on resident acuity. From a national perspective, the average Case Mix is 0.37, showing that this state is slightly lower than the national average. The reported LPN Staffing Hours per Resident per day is 0.87 noted as Quality Metric VOCHRD. This is on par with the national data of 0.87; therefore, this facility meets the percentage of LPN staffing hours as compared with the national average. According to the Quality Metric performance indicators for the last cycle, QM 401 (the percentage of long-stay residents whose need for help with daily activities increased) shows 11.1% of all long-stay residents need for help with activities has increased. Compared with the national average, which is 14.5%, this figure is lower. QM 453 (the percentage of long-stay residents with pressure sore injury) is 8.2%, compared with the national average of 7.3%. Overall, these last 2 sets of data reflect a poor performance for the management of pressure sore injury and an on par performance for the care of residents needing help with activities.

Nursing: Nursing Care Goals and Interventions

Post hip repair surgery, the nursing interventions centered on activities to assist with ambulation and to progress Mrs G's mobility within her room and eventually on the unit. When in bed, nurses turned and positioned Mrs G every 4 hours around the clock. Because of the recent hip fracture, Mrs G's care centered on assessment for postoperative infection by monitoring her cognitive status and vital signs. Nurses provided guidance in instruction for coughing and deep breathing exercises. Mrs G also was given anti-embolic stockings to prevent blood clots. The nurse reported a tar appearing black mark on her heel which was evaluated and determined to be a stage IV heel pressure sore with dry necrosis. The area was debrided with Santyl and monitored three times per week.

Health: Outcomes

For Mrs G, her ability to move independently was decreasing with an overall reduction in mobility. She developed the pressure injury. Two weeks postadmission to the LTC facility, Mrs G was noted to have nausea, vomiting, and an alteration in level of consciousness requiring an emergency room evaluation. Mrs G was diagnosed with sepsis and admitted to the hospital. In the hospital, she rapidly deteriorated, requiring intensive care unit monitoring. Within 24 hours Mrs G passed away with family at her bedside.

Using the quality metrics, or outcome indicators, areas of nursing practice that would be open to further investigation include: ambulation, skin integrity, and monitoring for infection. Another indicator of frailty, loss of weight,[18] was absent from the CASE study but also bears further investigation.

NURSING LEADERSHIP

To enact leadership in the area of quality and safety, nurses should be able to incorporate data-driven benchmarks to monitor system performance, evaluate the alignment of system data and comparative patient safety benchmarks, lead the analysis of actual errors, near misses, and potential situations that would impact safety, foster a culture of safety and respect.[19] Nurse leaders need to be familiar with the quality metrics listed on the CMS database, identify those that may reflect nursing care, master the ability to run reports from the database, and monitor these findings over time. While the CMS Quality Metrics are available for use by nurse managers in LTC facilities, how these can be aligned into benchmarks to establish industry standards and support comparison between individual facilities requires greater investment. We have illustrated that they can be used to benchmark around key conditions prevalent in the LTC context, in this CASE around frailty.

Nurses should lead the analysis of individual resident journeys, when poor outcomes including death, are experienced. Developing specialist skills in analytical techniques, such as those for root cause analysis,[20] position nurses working in the LTC sector well. We recommend that nurse leaders in LTC facilities undertake training in methodologies related to CASE analysis, to ensure that the issues are clearly identified. From this case study, a focus on nursing practices related to ambulation, skin integrity, monitoring for infection, and by implication, monitoring weight are worthy of further investigation. Follow-up investigation would require a review of practice, possible through audit or direct observation to fully understand any barriers and enablers in the care of residents who have been identified as frail. Here it would be very important to note which practice delivery models were most impactful in the LTC facility? For example, greater improvement in health outcomes may be noted from the use of patient-centered care practice delivery models. In the analysis of individual resident journeys, nursologists have a critical role, paving the way for thinking about the best venue for the delivery of nursing care. This is especially important in the LTC industry whereby older adults may spend their remaining years alongside professional nurses. Nursologists draw on existing conceptual models, such as Roy's Adaptation Model or Neuman's Systems Model, and/or other conceptual models and mid-range theories to shape how the person and their situation are viewed, ultimately influencing the delivery of nursing care.

Finally, fostering a culture of safety and respect is critical for continuous improvement.[21] Relationally focused leadership styles, such as transformational leadership,[22] individualized consideration,[23] and resonant leadership,[24] promote a positive workplace culture.[21] For nurse leaders in LTC facilities, it is important to mentor others in their professional growth and accountability, and influence and monitor intentional change to ensure continuous organizational improvement.

Specifically, in relation to the CASE study, a root cause analysis would consider:

- Person: How frailty is recognized and managed. The use of a frailty scale[25] for early recognition of frailty in the LTC setting is worthy of further investigation.
- Environment: Ask about the culture of care and safety, nurse staffing, and skill-mix, such as the number of RN hours per resident day, and resident census. Evidence suggests that higher levels or nurse staffing are correlated with higher

quality of care.[26] Skill mix in facilities that had higher numbers of RNs compared with licensed practical nurses had significantly lower rehospitalization and ED use.[27]

- Nursing care: Are nursing staff able to meet the care requirements for the residents? For example, missing meals is one example of a gap in practice[28] that requires monitoring. Audits or direct observations of practice may be required to gather further information about the delivery of nursing care.

Nurse experts have long noted these dynamic factors which influence the practice delivery model include, among others, a supportive practice environment, that is, adequate RN coverage and appropriate staffing according to resident's needs, and provision of RNs who possess geriatric nursing and leadership competencies.[29] The COVID-19 pandemic has revealed, however, shortcomings and "longstanding internal problems in nursing homes and the weak structures and policies that are meant to protect residents," further eroding supportive practice environments.[29] Two of the quintessential elements needed to deliver quality care, such as identifying and using an effective practice delivery model and utilization of a conceptual model by nurses, to care for frail residents, are often under the direct control of nurse managers and leaders.

SUMMARY

How nurse leaders can use Mitchell's Health Outcome conceptual framework to guide the identification of practice gaps and associated key leadership competencies to enact practice change for improved quality of care for people experiencing frailty was outlined in this article. Using an established conceptual framework, key nurse-sensitive outcome measures from the CMS Quality Metrics database were used to identify potential gaps in nursing care. Nurse leadership, in relation to quality improvement in LTC settings, should focus on how to incorporate data-driven benchmarks to monitor system performance, develop a structured approach for team analysis of actual errors, near misses, and potential situations that would impact safety, and foster a culture of safety and respect.[19]

CLINICS CARE POINTS

- Identify practice gaps in care to improve quality resident outcomes.

- Assess and mitigate contextual factors within the nursing meta-paradigm of human being, health, environment, and nursing goals which impact older adult health outcomes.

- Analyze the way by which nursing is delivered best to older adults' in your facility through various practice delivery models: primary or team nursing, patient centered care.

- Utilize quality metric indicators among older adult residents to determine the delivery of quality care.

ACKNOWLEDGMENT

The authors wish to thank Dr Jacqueline Fawcett for her thoughtful guidance as this article evolved.

DISCLOSURE

The authors have no financial or commercial conflicts associated with the information presented in this article.

REFERENCES

1. Centers for Disease Control and Prevention. Fast Stats: Nursing Home Care. Available at: https://www.cdc.gov/nchs/fastats/nursing-home-care.htm. Accessed on June 13, 2021.
2. Centers for Medicare and Medicaid Services. Quality Measures. Available at: https://www.cms.gov/Medicare/Quality-Initiatives-Patient-Assessment-Instruments/QualityMeasures. Accessed on June 13, 2021.
3. Agency for Healthcare Research and Quality. Types of healthcare quality measures. 2015. Available at: https://www.ahrq.gov/talkingquality/measures/types.html. Accessed on June 13, 2021.
4. American Nurses Association. Nursing: scope and standards of practice. 3rd edition. Silver Spring: American Nurses Association; 2015.
5. Fawcett J. Applying conceptual models of nursing: quality improvement, Research, and practice. New York: Springer Publishing; 2016.
6. Vetrano DL, Palmer K, Marengoni A, et al. Joint Action ADVANTAGE WP4 Group. Frailty and multimorbidity: a systematic review and meta-analysis. J Gerontol A Biol Sci Med Sci 2019;74(5):659–66.
7. Hanlon P, Nicholl BI, Jani BD, et al. Frailty and pre-frailty in middle-aged and older adults and its association with multimorbidity and mortality: a prospective analysis of 493 737 UK Biobank participants. Lancet Public Health 2018;3(7):e323–32.
8. Bagshaw SM, Stelfox HT, Johnson JA, et al. Long-term association between frailty and health-related quality of life among survivors of critical illness: a prospective multicenter cohort study. Crit Care Med 2015;43(5):973–82.
9. Kanwar A, Singh M, Lennon R, et al. Frailty and health-related quality of life among residents of long-term care facilities. J Aging Health 2013;25(5):792–802.
10. Gray-Miceli D, Rogowski J, de Cordova PB, et al. A framework for delivering nursing care to older adults with COVID-19 in nursing homes. Public Health Nurs 2021;00:1–17.
11. Personal communication with Dr Jacqueline Fawcett, June, 15, 2021.
12. Fawcett, J., & Richman, K. (2020, December 8). Primary care, primary nursology, and the attending nursologist: connections to nursology conceptual models and theories. Available at: https://nursology.net/2020/12/08/primary-care-primary-nursology-and-the-attending-nursologist-connections-to-nursology-conceptual-models-and-theories/.
13. Wasfy JH, Zigler CM, Choirat C, et al. Readmission rates after passage of the hospital readmissions reduction program: a pre-post analysis. Ann Intern Med 2017;166(5):324–31.
14. Bail K, Grealish L. Failure to maintain': a theoretical proposition for a new quality indicator of nurse care rationing for complex older people in hospital. Int J Nurs Stud 2016;63:146–61.
15. Clegg A, Young J, Iliffe S, et al. Frailty in elderly people. Lancet 2013;381(9868):752–62 [Erratum apperas in Lancet 2013;382(9901):1328].
16. Ouslander JG, Engstrom G, Reyes B, et al. Management of acute changes in condition in skilled nursing facilities. J Am Geriatr Soc 2018;66:2259–66.
17. Thornlow DK, Anderson R, Oddone E. Cascade iatrogenesis: factors leading to the development of adverse events in hospitalized older adults. Int J Nurs Stud 2009;46(11):1528–35.
18. Church S, Rogers E, Rockwood K, et al. A scoping review of the Clinical Frailty Scale. BMC Geriatr 2020;20(1):393.

19. American Association of Colleges of Nursing. The essentials: core competencies for professional nursing education. Washington (DC). 2021. Available at: https://www.aacnnursing.org/Education-Resources/AACN-Essentials. Accessed June 9, 2021.
20. Peerally MF, Carr S, Waring J, et al. The problem with root cause analysis. BMJ Qual Saf 2017;26(5):417–22.
21. Cummings GG, Tate K, Lee S, et al. Leadership styles and outcome patterns for the nursing workforce and work environment: A systematic review. Int J Nurs Stud 2018;85:19–60.
22. Bass BM, Avolio BJ. Improving organizational effectiveness through transformational leadership. London (United Kingdom): SAGE Publications; 1994.
23. Avolio BJ, Bass BM, Jung DI. Re-examining the components of transformational and transactional leadership using the multifactor leadership questionnaire. J Occup Organizational Psychol 1999;72(4):441–62.
24. Goleman D, Boyatzis R, McKee A. The new leaders: transforming the art of Leadership into the Science of Results. London (United Kingdom): Little, Brown; 2002.
25. Church S, Rogers E, Rockwood K, et al. A scoping review of the Clinical Frailty-Scale. BMC Geriatr 2020;20(1):393.
26. Dellefield ME, Castle NG, McGilton KS, et al. The relationship between registered nurses and nursing home quality: an integrative review (2008-2014). Nurs Econ 2015;33(2):95–108, 116.
27. Yang BK, Carter MW, Trinkoff AM, et al. Nurse staffing and skill mix patterns in relation to resident care outcomes in US Nursing Homes. J Am Med Dir Assoc 2021;22(5):1081–7.e1.
28. Chaboyer W, Harbeck E, Lee BO, et al. Missed nursing care: an overview of reviews. Kaohsiung J Med Sci 2021;37(2):82–91.
29. Bakerjian D, Boltz M, Bowers B, et al. Expert nurse response to workforce recommendations made by the Coronavirus Commission for safety and quality in nursing homes. Nurs Outlook 2021. https://doi.org/10.1016/j.outlook.2021.03.017.

Nursing Leadership – Transforming the Work Environment in Nursing Homes

Mary Ellen Dellefield, PhD, RN, FAAN[a],*, Caroline Madrigal, PhD, RN[b]

KEYWORDS

- Nursing homes • Nursing • Care delivery • Work environment
- Information exchange • Management

KEY POINTS

- The nursing work environment is a useful construct for understanding nursing home quality from a system-level perspective.
- Variables included in the construct are modifiable and actionable for nurse leaders interested in advancing nursing home quality.
- For-profit ownership and the social regulatory framework significantly impact the work environment of nurses in nursing homes.

INTRODUCTION

Nursing services in the nursing home (NH) are best understood operationally and strategically using a systems-level perspective.[1,2] Multiple variables impact the clinical practice of an individual nurse, work groups, and NHs. Although complex and challenging to measure rigorously, a systems-level perspective enables one to consider the impact of nursing services on organizational performance and important quality indicators for individual residents, and society at large.[3]

The work environment of nurses is a construct based on a systems-level perspective that supports the examination of multiple dimensions of nursing work and how it is influenced by internal and external variables.[1,4] As part of the quality chasm series of the Institute of Medicine, now referred to as the National Academy of Medicine, it published the seminal report "Keeping Patients Safe: Transforming the Work Environment of Nurses" (2004) for which the nursing work environment of multiple settings, including NHs, was examined. Variables highlighted included management practices, workforce capability and development (eg, staffing), work design, and a culture of safety.[4] Although the goals of Magnet hospitals have focused for several years on

^a Department of Community Health Systems, School of Nursing, University of California, San Francisco, 2 Koret Way, San Francisco, CA 94143-0608, USA; ^b Center of Innovation in Longterm Services and Supports, Providence VA Medical Center, 830 Chalkstone Avenue, Providence, RI 02908, USA
* Corresponding author.
E-mail addresses: mary.dellefield@ucsf.edu; dellefield@aol.com

Nurs Clin N Am 57 (2022) 299–314
https://doi.org/10.1016/j.cnur.2022.02.008
0029-6465/22/Published by Elsevier Inc.
nursing.theclinics.com

the professional nursing work environments in acute care, comparatively little research has been conducted to describe and explain this construct in NH settings.[5]

The purposes of this article are to: describe and explain variables known to be associated with the work environment of nurses in NHs and summarize evidence-based best practices with the capacity to transform the work environment for nursing staff. These will be examined by reviewing: the definition of the construct; the history and characteristics of NHs in the United States as organizational entities; the nature of nursing work; the nursing skill mix and care delivery; evidence-based best practices used by nursing leaders to transform the nursing work environment; and recommendations for future research and advocacy.

Given the long and seemingly intractable quality problems endemic in the NH, despite years of social regulation and enforcement, examination of the work environment may help nurses to understand why delivering quality care in this setting is so challenging.[6] It will provide evidence-based nursing leadership practices that may have the capacity to transform the work environment.[7] It will help members of interprofessional teams and society at large to better understand the extant internal and external system-level barriers that contribute to nursing's ongoing challenge in providing quality care in NHs.

NURSING WORK ENVIRONMENT

The construct of the nursing work environment is used to explain the link between an individual nurse's practice behaviors, the social environment or setting for which the work is performed, organizational performance, and resident outcomes.[1,4] Florence Nightingale first recognized the importance of the physical and social environment to promote health.[8] The nursing work environment was addressed in the IOM (2004) report by asserting that "the typical work environment of nurses is characterized by many serious threats to patient safety...These threats include basic components of all organizations—organizational management practices, workforce deployment practices, work design, and organizational culture" (p. 3).[4]

Although limited in numbers, studies have found that multiple aspects of NH operations must be addressed to promote a positive work environment. For example, it requires better staffing ratios, competitive compensation, less stressful workloads, and collaborative teamwork.[9] When staff feel they have a supportive work environment, they experience less stress, burnout, turnover, and poor health-related outcomes, as well as better job satisfaction.[10] Further, when a positive work environment is evident, residents experience fewer pressure ulcers, hospitalizations, and episodes of incontinence.[11] Temkin-Greener and colleagues (2009) posited that the work environment NH in NHs, when viewed as a measure of organizational performance, includes leadership; communication and coordination; and conflict management. These variables have an impact on staff cohesion and organizational performance, as measured by perceived work effectiveness.[1]

HISTORY AND CHARACTERISTICS OF NHs AS ORGANIZATIONS

NHs in the United States, as a component of the long-term care system, are uniquely complex. The dual legacy of social regulation and for-profit ownership of NHs has significantly impacted the quality of care and quality of life of residents, as well as the quality of the work environment.[4] A summary of the evolution of the NH provides context for our description of the NH work environment.

Institutional care has a rich history, beginning with the colonial establishment of almshouses or "poor houses" and church-affiliated rest homes which were privately run institutions for the most vulnerable older people.[12] Subsequently, the proprietary nature and early government involvement in NHs strongly influenced their evolution.[13] The Social Security Act of 1935 (Act of August 14, 1935) [H.R. 7260], provided states with money to help older adults in need of assistance. Other regulatory interventions influenced the evolution of the NH, including the 1954 Hill-Burton Act that stimulated the construction of NHs.[14] For example, in 1954 the majority of NHs, 86% were proprietary, 10% were voluntary, and 4% were public.[12]

The governmental response to the needs of older people was expanded in the 1965 landmark Medicare and Medicaid legislation that established a federally regulated NH industry.[14] This entitlement program attracted private industry to continue to invest and develop NHs. Of the 15,600 US NHs operating in 2016%, 69.3% of NH had for-profit ownership, the majority of which were operated by large corporations.[15] Increasingly, managed care plans and alternate reimbursement sources are influencing the NH industry.[16] Complex financial structures have been developed to decrease NH risk of litigation and use them primarily as real estate investments, rather than health care facilities.[17] All the while, the taxpayer is financing these arrangements through the government reimbursement system.

The Medicare and Medicaid NH Regulatory Framework

The content of regulations has been influenced by the historic Institute of Medicine report - *Improving Quality of Care in Nursing Homes (1986)*[18]; the *Nursing Home Reform Act (1986)*,[19] and 2016 standards of practice (ie, Conditions of Participation (CoP) issued by the Centers for Medicare and Medicaid Services).[20] The fundamental goal of the regulatory framework is to ensure resident safety and protect civil rights.[19] Although commonly thought of as defining the baseline for care, we argue that the regulatory requirements define excellence in care. For example, the stated goal is to help the resident achieve the highest practicable level of well-being.[19] It is the mandated requirements for investment in human capital that are baseline standards.

We recognize that government is legitimately interested in supporting quality care in the least costly way. Similarly, NH investors and shareholders' self-interests are returned on the investment and societal recognition of service quality (eg, 5-star ratings and receipt of deficiency citations associated with no actual harm to residents). However, this long-standing relationship between the NH industry and government reimbursement creates a perception of conflict of interest, as the government is challenged with the dual role of payor and regulator.

Given the nature of the existing NH industry, it is in the individual nurse's self-interest to acknowledge the inherent tensions that exist in this practice setting. These include the dominance of for-profit NHs in a fundamentally labor-intensive service industry. For example, researchers have demonstrated that not-for-profit NHs provide a higher level of a range of quality indicators to residents than for-profit NHs.[21] Arguably, the detailed regulation of nursing practice in the NH has diminished critical thinking skills of nurses, working in an environment that focuses primarily on the documentation of regulatory compliance.[22,23] Sadly, the nurse remains in a relatively vulnerable and powerless position in relation to NH owners and corporations.[24]

THE NATURE OF NURSING WORK

Sociologists have defined work as anything that a person undertakes, whether physical or mental exertion, for the purposes of being productive in meeting human needs.[25] Nursing practice, whether clinical or administrative in nature, is a type of work. Traditionally, nursing has been viewed as "a calling"—something that transcended merely working or having a job. At its core, nursing work involves social relationships with care recipients, patients, focusing on "knowing" the person as more than an object of clinical practice and procedures.[26] See **Box 1** for a summary of the characteristics of nursing work.

Florence Nightingale and Virginia Henderson were the pre-eminent leaders of nursing as a discipline and applied science.[7,27] The discipline of nursing has been defined by the domains of the person, health, (the act of) nursing, and the environment, both physical and psychosocial.[28] In essence, nursing responds to the biological, psychological, social, and spiritual dimensions of personhood. Other essential attributes include nursing's wholistic perspective of the person, the importance of individualized care; continuity of care over time; the impact of the practice context, and the temporal relationship with residents, on nursing practice. See **Box 2** for classic quotations from Nightingale and Henderson about the nature of nursing work.[7,27]

Nursing work may also be categorized as direct and indirect care.[29,30] Both are equally important.[31] Direct care includes assessment, giving medications/treatments, assisting with activities of daily living. Most of the direct care is performed by NAs/CNAs, ostensibly under the supervision of licensed nursing staff. Direct care includes activities of daily living, such as bathing, eating, walking, and using a toilet. Indirect care involves care provided on behalf of the resident, but away from them; it is focused on maintenance of the care environment.[30,31] Indirect care is typically performed by licensed staff [for example, registered nurses (RNs) and licensed vocational/practical nurses (LVNs/LPNs)]. See **Box 3** for a list of typical direct and indirect care nursing activities performed by licensed staff.

Box 1
Characteristics of nursing work in NHs

Applied science

Caring activities

Complex and multidimensional

Direct and indirect care

Historically hierarchical and rule-bound

Includes emotional labor

Labor intensive

Linked with female gender identity

Not observable

Observable

Predictable and unpredictable work

Regulated

Routine and nonroutine care

Standardized and individualized

Task oriented in resource-restricted environment

Temporally and contextually dependent

Undervalued

Visible and invisible

Box 2
The work of nursing: Florence Nightingale and Virginia Henderson

Florence Nightingale
"(Nursing) has been limited to signify little more than the administration of medicines and the application of poultices. It ought to signify the proper use of fresh air, light, warmth, cleanliness, quiet, and the proper selection and administration of diet—all at the least expense of vital power to the patient."
"For it may safely be said, not that the habit of ready and correct observation will by itself make us useful nurses, but that without it we shall be useless with all our devotion."

Virginia Henderson
"Health workers with less than professional preparation and people not classified as health workers but with special life experiences may be able to give certain kinds of help that most physicians and nurses either cannot give or are not interested in giving."
"The nursing process has served a useful purpose. However, if it is synonymous with problem-solving in the service of the client, it is no more peculiar to nursing than to medicine, dentistry, social work, or physiotherapy....It fails to stress the value of collaboration of health professionals and particularly the importance of developing the self-reliance of clients."

Study findings of how licensed nurses have used their time in direct and indirect care are instructive. For example, Burgio and colleagues (1990) observed nursing staff behaviors over a 37-month period and reported RNs used 48% of their time performing direct care and 52% of their time on indirect care processes.[32] Cardona and colleagues (1997) observed RN, LVN, and CNA work activities in a 60-bed VA operated NH care unit. They determined that RNs spent 34% of their time in direct care processes and 66% on indirect care processes.[33] Research findings of Hall and O'Brien-Pallas (2000) suggested that a higher level of RN involvement in direct care, and increased focus on the importance of direct care work, may benefit both nursing staff collectively, and residents.[34]

In more recent studies, Horn and colleagues (2005) targeted RN time spent in direct care processes how it affected PU incidence in at-risk NH residents, hospitalizations, urinary tract infections, weight loss, catheterizations, deterioration in ADL

Box 3
Direct and indirect care performed by licensed nurses

Direct care
  Activities related to care transitions (admission, transfer, death, changes in condition)
  Activities of daily living
  Clinical assessment, observation, surveillance
  Communication/information exchange among IDT or nursing staff
  Infection control
  Medications/treatments
  Resident/family communications/meetings

Indirect care
  Budget/finance
  Hiring, personnel matters
  Nursing staff and interdepartmental meetings
  Program development (implementing new regulations; policies and procedures)
  QAPI
  Staffing
  Supervision/management
  Survey preparation
  Training/education

performance, and greater use of oral nutritional supplements. More RN direct care hours per resident day (HPRD) were associated with fewer negative outcomes.[35] Using work sample of RNs working on the day shift in one NH, Dellefield, Harrington, and Kelly reported that RNs spent 59% of their time on indirect care, with scant observation of direct care focused on pressure ulcer prevention.[36] Although there is evidence that some care outcomes are improved when more direct care is provided by licensed nurses, the current reality is that it is not economically feasible to increase NH nurses' direct care time, given the extant reimbursement system.[35,37]

It is noteworthy that the work design and related management practices comprising the nursing work environment refer largely to indirect care.[1,34,37] Indirect care is important, although the nursing profession has undervalued indirect care, to its detriment.[31] For example, indirect care is frequently mischaracterized as generic administrative work. It is essential that RNs working in NHs understand the value of their work as indirect care to support the provision of direct care. See **Box 3**.

With the welcomed advancement and increased presence of advanced practice nurses (APNs) in the NH, it is essential that APNs understand and respect the role of the nurse leader, manager, and supervisor in performing indirect care.[38] Although indirect care may involve activities related to the NHs infrastructure, such as scheduling, evaluations, and payroll, their value is understood as both a means to the end of creating a safe and healthy work and care environment. The supportive work environment created by competent nurse leaders has been shown to be significantly associated with higher job satisfaction among RNs working in NHs.[11,39]

Because of its complex nature, measuring nursing work is challenging. Researchers have used a variety of methods to measure nursing work, including, direct observation, chart reviews, staff self-report, time studies, work sampling, and selected instruments summarized in a US Department of Health & Human Services, US Department of Labor report (2005).[40–44]

NURSING SKILL MIX

The nursing skill mix is an important component of nursing work. It refers to differences in the level of education and certification among nursing staff, comprised of RNs, LVNs/LPNs, and NAs/CNAs. RNs and LVNs/LPNs are commonly referred to as licensed staff.[4] The percentage of each type of licensed staff in the NH workforce differs significantly. Five percent of all RNs in the United States work in NHs, whereas 13% of all licensed vocational/practical nurses' work in NHs.[45] LPNs/LVNs function as medication and treatment nurses; charge/supervisory nurses; and contribute their clinical findings to the RAI/Minimum Data Set, a standardized assessment used by all US NHs receiving reimbursement from CMS. LVNs/LPNs also commonly function as directors of staff development and infection control nurses.

As the rubric of "licensed nurses" suggests, the NH industry has used RNs and LVNs/LPNs interchangeably since 1965; distinctions between practice roles have been limited.[46,47] As an economic strategy, this is known as a "perfect" substitute." That is, the quality of something considered as a "perfect substitute" is the same as that being substituted, except that it may be purchased at a lower cost.[48] Put another way, there is nothing that the RN contributes that the LVN/LPN cannot equally contribute. This approach meets federal staffing requirements but significantly limits the opportunity for RNs to demonstrate their capacity to add value to the nursing workforce because of their education and expertise in care coordination and surveillance.[49]

The actual implementation of the Resident Assessment Instrument (RAI)/Minimum Data Set (MDS) Nurse Coordination role is arguably the best illustration of the clinical consequences of using "licensed" nurses as the Medicare/Medicaid federal regulatory language. The regulation states that the RAI/MDS must be conducted or coordinated (or both) by an RN who signs and certifies the completion of the MDS and the RAPS.[19] If the RN is completing the MDS then their signature is certifying the accuracy of the assessment. However, if the RN is coordinating the MDS process, and other clinicians are completing specific sections, the RN signature certifies only the completion of the MDS process. Therefore, it is possible for LVN/LPNs to complete the MDS and care planning decision, sign to certify its accuracy, and obtain an RN signature to certify the completion of the MDS and RAP assessment process. The result is that LVNs/LPNs throughout the nation may routinely be practicing outside of their scope of practice.[46,47] There also is no requirement that the RAI/MDS licensed nurses must be certified as competent in the MDS process.[19] This is problematic, given the complexity and dynamic nature of the RAI process.

Since the 1940s, use of the nursing process, the foundational intervention associated with the RAI process, has been identified as the unique domain of those RNs educated in university settings, as opposed to a hospital or community college.[50] However, most RNs in NHs have either associates degrees or diplomas. Limited structural incentives exist for RNs working in NHs to attain higher education (ie, BSN or graduate-level degree).[51] Further, individual states have unique nursing practice acts, licensed vocational/practical nurse, and nursing assistant certifications.[52] This structural barrier exists in addition to the use of LVNs as perfect substitutes for RNs in NHs.

In spite of this widespread substitution of LVNs for RNs, studies have demonstrated that higher levels of RN staffing are associated with preferred clinical outcomes, such as reduced rehospitalizations; fewer pressure ulcers; lower restraint use; fewer deficiency citations; decreased mortality; lower NA and RN turnover; and decreased incidence of urinary tract infections.[48] In 2021, researcher reported that NHs with a high-RN cluster had the lowest rehospitalization and ED visit rates, whereas NHs with a high cluster of LPN staffing had the highest rehospitalization and ED visit rates among the sample. Although RN and LPN/LVN duties may overlap in facilities, the researchers suggested that LPNs/LVNs "may not be prepared for nursing duties that require greater clinical reasoning, such as resident assessment, evaluation, delegation, and supervision of unlicensed personnel." (p. 1082).[52] Further study and consideration of the nursing skill mix is needed.

SUPERVISION AND MANAGEMENT OF THE NURSING SKILL MIX

Clinical supervision is defined as real-time direction, oversight, and exchange of clinical information, or feedback.[53] Nursing supervisory practices in NHs have been described as inadequate; they have been associated with poor clinical outcomes, including increased staff turnover, reduced retention among nursing staff, using rule bound and hierarchical management approaches.[54–56] Chronic turnover adds to the burden of nurse leaders in providing continuity of care, establishing, and sustaining best practices, and persistent need for senior staff to provide orientation and mentorship. Descriptive study findings have reported evidence of flawed supervisory and managerial approaches used in NHs. For example, supervisors or charge nurses reported that nursing assistants have completed certification programs and ought to routinely perform their jobs without oversight or supervision.[57] Supervisors or charge nurses did not feel empowered as managers and perceived that they had no need for management skills.

Sadly, the staff member closest to the resident, the NA/CNA, and the provider of the most intimate resident care, has been the least respected. Arguably, this is demonstrated by the NH industry's persistent failure to address the issue of nursing assistant turnover, and the perception that "bed and body" nursing care requires little skill. In essence, it demonstrates a devaluation of basic nursing care.[58] The recent trend toward NA/CNA self-empowerment and respect within nursing services suggests that some professional nurses have been remiss in recognizing the essential role of the nursing assistant.[59,] This perspective may also suggest that the NA/CNA's work has come to be somewhat disconnected from the licensed nurse's work and practice.

One limitation of an unsupportive practice environment is that nursing staff may experience limited professional agency. Anderson and colleagues at Duke University - Center for Aging and Human Development has focused on the nursing agency. For example, agency is enhanced when all nursing staff experience involvement in decision-making.[60–62] Nursing staff are challenged to integrate a social and medical model of care in the contemporary NH. In understanding a resident's preferences, in knowing the resident, the nursing staff must respond to the resident's preferred model of care. A shared sense of meaning of the work of the nursing staff, its value, and impact on resident life is essential to achieve this.[22,23]

LEADERSHIP BEST PRACTICES

Researchers have demonstrated that NHs foster healthy communication between licensed nurses and certified nursing assistants, and collaborative clinical problem-solving produce optimal care experiences for residents. For example, coaching supervision provides an evidence-based alternative to traditional hierarchical supervision.[63] The characteristics of coaching supervision are identical to those promulgated in culture change initiatives, patient safety programs, just culture, pressure ulcer prevention strategies, and high-reliability organizations.

While the nurse leader and RN are responsible for the comprehensive assessment of the resident, establishment, and implementation of the plan of care, NA/CNAs could play an essential role in the development of a feasible and effective care plan. Historically, there has been a tendency for RNs to discount the data collection and observational skills of NA/CNAs, thus diminishing their sense of worth and value to the nursing service.[49] To promote a sense of effective participation in decision making and empowerment, certified nursing assistants will benefit from knowing clear parameters in which their problem-solving, and judgment are exercised, as well as the requirements of their reporting relationship to the supervisory staff. See **Table 1** for a summary of evidence-based best leadership practices.[53–55,64,65]

Many organizations and projects provide examples of the best way forward. These include efforts by the John A. Hartford Foundation, Leading Age, American Association of Post-Acute Care Nursing (AAPACN), innovative nurse residency programs, including the LVN LEAD program,[66] advocacy for the certification of directors of nursing,[67] higher quality standards for nurse educators employed by NHs, and effective partnerships with paraprofessional groups, such as PHI,[63] working to advance the professionalism of NAs and CNAs. The ANCC Pathways to Excellence program provides an excellent resource for nurse leaders.[68]

RESEARCH FRAMEWORKS USED TO SUPPORT LEADERSHIP BEST PRACTICES

To fully appreciate evidence-based best practices associated with the work environment of nurses in NHs, it is important to have an awareness of the conceptual frameworks used by researchers. These are used to demonstrate how variables interact with one another to support or inhibit a healthy work environment. Frameworks include: Donabedian's quality framework,[69] complexity theory,[60–62] contingency theory,[70] and scarcity theory.[71,72]

Table 1	
Best nursing leadership and managerial practices in NHs	
Reference	Approach
Eaton, 2000[54]	High quality leadership & management; respecting & valuing staff, especially paraprofessionals; positive human resource practices; sufficient staff; social investment in staff with social policy component.
Harahan, 2003[78]	Clear expectations; all nursing staff seen as problem-solvers and decision-makers; Two-way accountability with mutual Respect; use of mentoring & role modeling; career advancement; strong & visible DON involved with resident care.
Dellefield, 2008[53]	Programs: ACT NOW; WIN An STEP UP; Growing Strong Roots; Coaching Supervision Curriculum (PHI); LEAP; CNA enrichment programs; consistent assignments; electronic documentation.
Siegel, Young, H.M., Mitchell, P.H., Shannon, S.E.,2008[79]	Nurse leaders require management competencies in working in complex organizational environment.
Toles, M.T. & Anderson, R.A, 2011[64]	Manage relationships between managers and staff; staff participation in decision-making; work designs that foster staff interactions; combine relationship-oriented management and evidence-based clinical practices.
Corazzini, K., Twersky, J, White, Heidi K., Buhr, G.T., McConnell, E.S., Weiner, M., Colon-Emeric, C.S, 2014[65]	Themes associated with culture change & an Adaptive Leadership Framework: relationships; standards and expectations; motivation and vision; workload; respect of personhood; physical environment.

Several researchers have used Donabedian's quality framework to support NH studies. Donabedian posited that quality is a complex and multidimensional construct. It includes dimensions of structure, process, and outcome, each of which may have technical and interpersonal aspects. Quality may only be measured indirectly, using measures or indicators associated with each dimension.

Complexity theory has been used extensively by Anderson and colleagues to describe and explain nursing staff behaviors in NHs and its system-level operations.[60–62] A basic tenet of contingency theory is that organizational outcomes are determined primarily by the fit among the organizations' structure, tasks (eg, jobs), and its operating context. Core concepts include the work task itself and its relationship to the environment. The concept of work is fundamental to the contingency model of organization and management.[70] Most recently, the political and economic theory of scarcity has been used to explain how In nursing practice, time scarcity stimulates a decision-making process, known as clinical prioritization or implicit rationing. As nurse staffing shortages have become both a national and international issue, nurse researchers are using scarcity theory to better understand what is occurring at the point of care because of limited time, staffing, or skill mix.[71,72]

CARE DELIVERY

How care is delivered is affected by several variables, some of which include the quality and quantity of human capital, the physical layout of the NH itself, and the degree to which computer technology is integrated into the work flow of staff. The composition of the nursing workforce has a significant impact on how care may be delivered because members of the nursing skill mix have different roles and competencies. Each member of the skill mix has their specific job description and defined activities that may or may not be consistent with the scope of practice regulations in individual states.[73,74]

Traditional methods of nursing care delivery have included primary care, functional nursing, and team nursing delivered over 3 work shifts.[4] Although the rubric of teams is commonly used in the NH literature, functional nursing dominates.[4] Given limited federal staffing requirements, regulators have given little guidance on the actual care delivery system, other than focus on the use of the nursing process and interprofessional assessments.[20]

The basic function of a care delivery system in an NH is to provide the mechanism by which nursing care, in all its dimensions, is provided as a service to residents. The service is, by definition, interactive in nature. Besides supporting the delivery of physical care, the care delivery system may be viewed as the mechanism by which accurate and timely information is exchanged among staff and residents. Although some point to the importance of the nursing process, the care plan, and care planning as the dominant means of information exchange in NH care delivery, there is limited evidence that this occurs or is the most feasible way of exchanging information.[50,75] A basic challenge in designing a care delivery system is that it needs to include approaches to information exchange that are feasible and sustainable among all nursing staff and interprofessional team members.[76] Use of the work environment construct provides an opportunity to look information exchange within the NH care delivery system in a more sophisticated way.

Information exchange among NAs and CNAs consists primarily of ongoing communication with licensed nurses, communications with residents, meaningful participation in care conferences, and exchange of observations during change in shift report or rounding. Specifically, staff shortages and turnover are persistent barriers to effective information exchange within the nursing skill mix. An anecdotal practice that occurs in some for-profit NHs is the elimination of change in shift report or overlap between shifts of nursing assistants. This is a cost-cutting strategy that may result in limited information exchange among NAs and CNAs.

A distinctive aspect of information exchange affecting RNs in their leadership roles is that they need to use the information contained in national information systems. These include ongoing regulatory mandates from CMS, the CASPER (Certification and Survey Provider Enhanced Reports), QIES (Quality Improvement and Evaluation System), and ASPEN (Automated Survey Process Environment). As of May 2021, these databases were consolidated and accessible through the Internet Quality Improvement and Evaluation Center (iQIES).[77] A better understanding of operational opportunities related to NA/CNA and licensed nurse information exchange has the potential to support more effective supervisory, managerial, and care delivery practices.

FUTURE RESEARCH AND ADVOCACY

The challenges faced by nurses working in NHs are substantial, as reflected in the complexity of the notion of nursing work and the work environment itself. The hope is that nurse researchers will continue to build on the body of research that has already been developed to enhance our understanding of our work as nurses and our work environment. Unlike other providers in NHs, nurses are the only professionals who provide a 24-h presence in facilities. This alone provides us with a unique perspective that needs to be honored and incorporated into future for the reformation of the NH and long-term care health care system. Greater investment in research dollars is needed to better understand the complex interactions of variables included in the work environment construct and resident outcomes.

The work environment is a modifiable construct associated with improving the quality of NH care. To achieve desired changes, a respectful understanding of the contributions made by all nursing staff is needed, regardless of their level of education and skill. The care delivery system must maximize the contributions of all members of the nursing skill mix. Research on better understanding the unique contributions of direct and indirect nursing care needs to be supported. A strong and clear understanding of the value that the nursing service adds to the interprofessional team is very much needed.

The experience with the pandemic has demonstrated how vulnerable NHs are operational. The solutions are complex and do not involve any one thing. We are the professionals challenged to mesh the medical and social models of care needed to sustain both quality of care and quality of life to NH residents. Nurse leaders have the capacity to contribute to the transformation of the nursing work environment if they embrace a systems-level understanding of the NH.

We suggest that the linchpin of them all is arguably better staffing and higher wages and benefits. This will provide a basic context in which other issues of care delivery, workforce development, and advancement of safety culture may advance. Unfortunately, addressing this will involve an investment of society's resources to solve problems that clearly cannot be solved by regulation alone.

SUMMARY

The nursing work environment is a complex construct. It involv es Johnson A, Guillano JA, Bowers B, Stone R. (2003) clinical and managerial practices, workforce development that includes staffing and skill mix, the regulatory, and reimbursement context in which work is performed. It is helpful to remember that "the typical work environment of nurses is characterized by many serious threats to patient safety...These threats include.... organizational management practices, workforce deployment practices, work design, and organizational culture" (p. 3).[4] Our challenge is to continue to provide nursing leadership to positively impact this construct through practice, research, and scholarship.

CLINICS CARE POINTS

- The nursing work environment contains potential threats to patient safety.
- Nurse leaders must have an in-depth understanding of historic trends in nursing home ownership and regulation.

DISCLOSURE

The authors have nothing to disclose. This research did not receive any specific grant from funding agencies in the public, commercial, or not-for-profit sectors. This work was partially supported by Nursing and Patient Care Services, VA San Diego Healthcare System and the Center of Innovation in Long-term Services and Supports at the Providence VA Medical Center via the Office of Academic Affiliation's Advanced Fellowship in Health Services Research (Dr C. Madrigal). The views expressed in this article are those of the authors and do not necessarily reflect the position or policy of the Department of Veterans Affairs or the United States government.

REFERENCES

1. Temkin-Greener H, Zheng N, Katz P, et al. Measuring work environment and performance in nursing homes. Med Care 2009;47(4):482–91.
2. Temkin-Greener H, Zheng NT, Cai S, et al. Nursing home environment and organizational performance: association with deficiency citations. Med Care 2010; 48(4):357–64.
3. Wei H, Sewell KA, Woody G, et al. The state of the science of nurse work environments in the United States: a systematic review. Int J Nurs Sci 2018;5(3):287–300.
4. Institute of Medicine (US). Committee on the Work Environment for Nurses and Patient Safety. In: Page A, editor. Keeping patients safe: transforming the work environment of nurses. Washington, DC: National Academies Press (US); 2004. p. 65–224.
5. Park SH, Gass S, Boyle DK. Comparison of Reasons for Nurse Turnover in Magnet® and Non-Magnet Hospitals. J Nurs Adm 2016;46(5):284–90.
6. Grabowski DC. Strengthening nursing home policy for the postpandemic world : how can we improve residents' health outcomes and experiences? New York: The Commonwealth Fund; 2020.
7. Schalk DM, Bijl ML, Halfens RJ, et al. Interventions aimed at improving the nursing work environment: a systematic review. Implement Sci 2010;5:34.
8. Davies R. 'Notes on nursing: what it is and what it is not'. (1860): by Florence Nightingale. Nurse Educ Today 2012;32(6):624–6.
9. Lapane KL, Hughes CM. Considering the employee point of view: perceptions of job satisfaction and stress among nursing staff in nursing homes. J Am Med Dir Assoc 2007;8(1):8–13.
10. Zúñiga F, Ausserhofer D, Hamers JP, et al. Are staffing, work environment, work stressors, and rationing of care related to care workers' perception of quality of care? A Cross-Sectional Study. J Am Med Dir Assoc 2015;16(10):860–6.
11. White EM, Aiken LH, Sloane DM, et al. Nursing home work environment, care quality, registered nurse burnout and job dissatisfaction. Geriatr Nurs 2020; 41(2):158–64.
12. Michaels D. American nursing history: history of nursing homes in America-From the Almshouse to Person-Centered Homes. 2020. Available at: https:// static1squarespect.com. Accessed June 20, 2021.
13. Vladeck BC Unloving care: the nursing home tragedy. Polit Sci Q 1981. https:// doi.org/10.2307/2149702.
14. Morford TG. Nursing home regulation: history and expectations. Health Care Financ Rev Annu Suppl 1989;129–32.
15. Kohn NA, Geo LJ. Nursing homes, COVID-19 and the consequences of regulatory failure. Georgetown Law. Available at: https://www.law.georgetown.edu/georgetown-law-journal/glj-online. Accessed June 23, 2021;110(online 1).
16. Kingsley DE, Harrington C. COVID-19 had little financial impact on publicly traded nursing home companies. J Am Geriatr Soc 2021;69(8):2099–102.
17. Edelman T. Special Report: nursing facilities have received billions of dollars in direct financial and non-financial support during coronavirus pandemic. Washington (DC): Center for Medicare Advocacy; 2021. Available at: https:// medicareadvocacy.org/report-snf-financial-support-during-covid/.

18. Institute of Medicine (US). Committee on the Adequacy of Nursing Staff in Hospitals and Nursing Homes. In: Wunderlich GS, Sloan F, Davis CK, editors. Nursing staff in hospitals and nursing homes: is it adequate? Washington, DC: National Academies Press (US); 1996.

19. Omnibus Budget Reconciliation Act of 1987. H.R. 3545. Available at: https://www.congress.gov.bill/100th-congress/house-bill/3545. Accessed May 20, 2021.

20. Centers for Medicare and Medicaid Services. State operations manual, chapter 7 – survey and enforcement process for skilled nursing facilities and nursing facilities. 2018. Available at: https://www.cms.gov/Regulations-and-Guidance/Guidance/Manuals/downloads/som107c07.pdf. Accessed May 15, 2021.

21. Comondore VR, Devereaux PJ, Zhou Q, et al. Quality of care in for-profit and not-for-profit nursing homes: systematic review and meta-analysis. BMJ 2009;339: b2732.

22. Anderson RA, Ammarell N, Bailey D Jr, et al. Nurse assistant mental models, sensemaking, care actions, and consequences for nursing home residents. Qual Health Res 2005;15(8):1006–21.

23. Colón-Emeric CS, Plowman D, Bailey D, et al. Regulation and mindful resident care in nursing homes. Qual Health Res 2010;20(9):1283–94.

24. Kolanowski A, Cortes TA, Mueller C, et al. A call to the CMS: mandate adequate professional nurse staffing in nursing homes. Am J Nurs 2021;121(3):24–7.

25. Barnes RM. Motion and time study design and measurement of work. 7th edition. John Wiley & Sons; 1980.

26. May C. Nursing work, nurses' knowledge, and the subjectification of the patient. Sociol Health Illn 1992;14(4):472–87.

27. Halloran EJ. A Virginia Henderson reader: excellence in nursing. Springer Publishing Co.; 1996.

28. Nikfarid L, Hekmat N, Vedad A, et al. The main nursing metaparadigm concepts in human caring theory and Persian mysticism: a comparative study. J Med Ethics Hist Med 2018;11:6.

29. Department of Health, Education & Welfare, Division of Nursing. Methods for studying nurse staffing in a patient unit. DHEW Pub. No HRA 78-3. DHEW: Washington (DC).

30. Wolf Z. Direct and indirect care: defining domains of nursing practice. Int J Hum Caring 1997;1(3):43–52.

31. Allen D. The invisible work of nurses: hospitals, organization and healthcare. Oxford (UK), New York: Routedge; 2015.

32. Burgio LD, Engel BT, Hawkins A, et al. A descriptive analysis of nursing staff behaviors in a teaching nursing home: differences among NAs, LPNs, and RNs. Gerontologist 1990;30(1):107–12.

33. Cardona P, Tappen RM, Terrill M, et al. Nursing staff time allocation in long-term care: a work sampling study. J Nurs Adm 1997;27(2):28–36.

34. Hall LM, O'Brien-Pallas L. Redesigning nursing work in long-term care environments. Nurs Econ 2000;18(2):79–87.

35. Horn SD, Buerhaus P, Bergstrom N, et al. RN staffing time and outcomes of long-stay nursing home residents: pressure ulcers and other adverse outcomes are less likely as RNs spend more time on direct patient care. Am J Nurs 2005; 105(11):58–71.

36. Dellefield ME, Harrington C, Kelly A. Observing how RNs use clinical time in a nursing home: a pilot study. Geriatr Nurs 2012;33(4):256–63.

37. Montayre J, Montayre J. Nursing work in long-term care: an integrative review. J Gerontol Nurs 2017;43(11):41–9.

38. Gray-Miceli D, Rogowski J, de Cordova PB, et al. A framework for delivering nursing care to older adults with COVID-19 in nursing homes. Public Health Nurs 2021;38(4):610–26.

39. Choi J, Flynn L, Aiken LH. Nursing practice environment and registered nurses' job satisfaction in nursing homes. Gerontologist 2012;52(4):484–92.

40. Schnelle JF, Bates-Jensen BM, Chu L, et al. Accuracy of nursing home medical record information about care-process delivery: implications for staff management and improvement. J Am Geriatr Soc 2004;52(8):1378–83.

41. Leatt P, Schneck R. Nursing subunit technology: a replication. Adm Sci Q 1981; 26(2):225–36.

42. Leppa CJ. Measuring nursing work in long-term care. The reliability and validity of the Leatt Measure of Nursing Technology. J Gerontol Nurs 1999;25(10):40–5.

43. Centers for Medicare and Medicaid Services (CMS). Patient Driven Payment Model (PDPM). 2021. Available at: https://www.com.gov/pdpm. Accessed July 2, 2021.

44. Liefer KM, Harris-Kojetin L, Brannon D, et al. Measuring Long-term care work: a guide to selected instruments to examine direct care worker experiences and outcomes. US Department of Health & Human Services, US Department of Labor, Institute for the Future of Aging Services. 2005. Available at: http://aspe.hhs.gov/daltcp/reports/dcwguide.htm. Accessed June 2, 2021.

45. National Nursing Workforce Study NCSBN. 2021. Available at: https://www.ncsbn.org. Accessed August 3, 2021.

46. Corazzini KN, McConnell ES, Day L, et al. Differentiating scopes of practice in nursing homes: collaborating for care. J Nurs Regul 2015;6(1):43–9.

47. Mueller C, Duan Y, Vogelsmeier A, et al. Interchangeability of licensed nurses in nursing homes: perspectives of directors of nursing. Nurs Outlook 2018;66(6):560–9.

48. Dellefield ME, Castle NG, McGilton KS, et al. The relationship between registered nurses and nursing home quality: an integrative review (2008-2014). Nurs Econ 2015;33(2):95–116.

49. Dellefield ME, Madrigal CB, Verkaaik C, et al. Nursing surveillance and immediate jeopardy in Veteran Health Administration community living centers unannounced survey program 2018 to 2019. Nurs Outlook 2021;69(2):182–92.

50. Dellefield ME. Interdisciplinary care planning and the written care plan in nursing homes: a critical review. Gerontologist 2006;46(1):128–33.

51. Holle CL, Sundean LJ, Dellefield ME, et al. Examining the beliefs of skilled nursing facility directors of nursing regarding bsn completion and the impact of nurse leader education on patient outcomes. J Nurs Adm 2019;49(2):57–60.

52. Yang BK, Carter MW, Trinkoff AM, et al. Nurse staffing and skill mix patterns in relation to resident care outcomes in US Nursing Homes. J Am Med Dir Assoc 2021;22(5):1081–7.e1.

53. Dellefield ME. Best practices in nursing homes. Clinical supervision, management, and human resource practices. Res Gerontol Nurs 2008;1(3):197–207.

54. Eaton SC. Beyond 'unloving care': linking human resource management and patient care quality in nursing homes. Int J Hum Resource Manage 2000;11:591–616.

55. McGillis Hall L, McGilton KS, Krejci J, et al. Enhancing the quality of supportive supervisory behavior in long-term care facilities. J Nurs Adm 2005;35(4):181–7.

56. Bowers BJ, Esmond S, Jacobson N. Turnover reinterpreted-CNAs talks about why they leave. J Gerontol Nurs 2003;29(3):36–43.

57. Dellefield ME. Nursing staff descriptions of clinical supervision and management in Veterans Affairs-affiliated nursing homes. J Nurs Care Qual 2008;23(1):66–74.

58. Harris-Kojetin L, Lipson D, Fielding J, et al. Recent findings on frontline long-term care workers: a research synthesis 1999-2003. Institute for the Future of Aging Services; 2004.

59. Yeatts DE, Cready CM. Consequences of empowered CNA teams in nursing home settings: a longitudinal assessment. Gerontologist 2007;47(3):323–39.

60. Anderson RA, McDaniel RR Jr. RN participation in organizational decision making and improvements in resident outcomes. Health Care Manage Rev 1999; 24(1):7–16.

61. Anderson RA, Plowman D, Corazzini K, et al. Participation in decision making -testing a measure. Nurs Res Pract 2013;706842.

62. Anderson RA, Corazzini KN, McDaniel RR Jr. Complexity science and the dynamics of climate and communication: reducing nursing home turnover. Gerontologist 2004;44(3):378–88.

63. Paraprofessional Health Institute. Coaching supervison: introductory skills for supervisors in home and residential care. Paraprofessional Healthcare Institute; 2005.

64. Toles MT, Anderson RA. State of the science: relationship-oriented management practices in nursing homes. Nurs Outlook 2011;59(4):221–7.

65. Corazzini K, Twershy J, White HK, et al. Implementing culture change in nursing homes: an adaptive leadership framework. Gerontologist 2014;55(4):616–27.

66. Harahan MF, Sanders A, Stone RI, et al. Gerontological Nursing. Available at: https://doi.org/10.3928/00989134-20110302-01. Accessed January 22, 2021;37(6).

67. Siegel E, Mueller C, Anderson K, et al. The pivotal role of the director of nursing in nursing homes. J Nurs Care Qual 2010;34(2):119–21.

68. American Nurses Credentialling Center. Pathways to Excellence. Available at: Nursingworld.org/ancc.

69. Donabedian A. The role of outcomes in quality assessment and assurance. Qual Rev Bull 1992;11:356–60.

70. Zinn JS, Brannon D, Mor V, et al. A structure-technology contingency analysis of caregiving in nursing facilities. Health Care Mgmt Rev 2003;28(4):293–306.

71. Primc N. Dealing with scarcity of resources in nursing. The scope and limits of individual responsibility. Eur J Nsg Hist Ethics 2020. https://doi.org/10.25974/enhe2020-8en.

72. Papastavrou E, Andreou P, Efstathiou G. Rationing of nursing care and nurse-patient outcomes: a systematic review of quantitative studies. Int J Health Plann Manage 2014;29:3–25.

73. Fernandez R, Johnson M, Tran DT, et al. Models of care in nursing: a systematic review. Int J Evid Based Healthc 2012;10(4):324–37.

74. Havaei F, Dahinten VS, MacPhee M. Effect of nursing care delivery models on registered nurse o53utcomes. SAGE Open Nurs 2019;5. https://doi.org/10.1177/2377960819869088. 2377960819869088.

75. Dellefield ME, Corazzini K. Comprehensive care plan development using resident assessment instrument framework: past, present, and future practices. Healthcare (Basel) 2015;3(4):1031–53.

76. Georgiou A, Marks A, Braithwaite J, et al. Gaps, disconnections, and discontinuities-the role of information exchange in the delivery of quality long-term care. Gerontologist 2012;53(5):770–9.

77. Internet Quality Improvement and Evaluation System (iQIES) -QTSO. 2021. Available at: https://iqies.cms.gov. Accessed August 5, 2021.
78. Harahan MF, Kiefer K, Johnson A, et al. Addressing shortages in the direct care workforce: The recruitment and retention practices of California's not-for-profit nursing homes. Continuing Care Retirement Communities and Assisted Living Facilities 2003.
79. Siegel E, Young H, Mitchell P, et al. Nurse preparation and organizational support for supervision of unlicensed assistive personnel in nursing homes: A qualitative exploration. The Gerontologist 2008;48(4):453–63.

FURTHER READING

Stone R, Harahan M. Improving the long-term care workforce serving older adults. Health Affairs 2010;29(1).

Moving?

Make sure your subscription moves with you!

To notify us of your new address, find your **Clinics Account Number** (located on your mailing label above your name), and contact customer service at:

Email: journalscustomerservice-usa@elsevier.com

800-654-2452 (subscribers in the U.S. & Canada)
314-447-8871 (subscribers outside of the U.S. & Canada)

Fax number: 314-447-8029

Elsevier Health Sciences Division
Subscription Customer Service
3251 Riverport Lane
Maryland Heights, MO 63043

*To ensure uninterrupted delivery of your subscription, please notify us at least 4 weeks in advance of move.